T0315311

Infectious Diseases in Obstetrics and Gynecology

Editors

KEVIN A. AULT
ALISA B. KACHIKIS

OBSTETRICS AND GYNECOLOGY CLINICS OF NORTH AMERICA

www.obgyn.theclinics.com

Consulting Editor
WILLIAM F. RAYBURN

June 2023 • Volume 50 • Number 2

ELSEVIER

1600 John F. Kennedy Boulevard • Suite 1800 • Philadelphia, Pennsylvania, 19103-2899

http://www.theclinics.com

OBSTETRICS AND GYNECOLOGY CLINICS OF NORTH AMERICA Volume 50 Number 2
June 2023 ISSN 0889-8545, ISBN-13: 978-0-443-18205-1

Editor: Kerry Holland
Developmental Editor: Hannah Almira Lopez

Obstetrics and Gynecology Clinics (ISSN 0889-8545) is published quarterly by Elsevier Inc., 360 Park Avenue South, New York, NY 10010-1710. Months of issue are March, June, September, and December. Periodicals postage paid at New York, NY, and additional mailing offices. Subscription price per year is $355.00 (US individuals), $757.00 (US institutions), $100.00 (US students), $428.00 (Canadian individuals), $956.00 (Canadian institutions), $100.00 (Canadian students), $487.00 (international individuals), $956.00 (international institutions), and $225.00 (international students). To receive student/resident rate, orders must be accompanied by name of affiliated institution, date of term, and the signature of program/residency coordinator on institution letterhead. Orders will be billed at individual rate until proof of status is received. Foreign air speed delivery is included in all *Clinics* subscription prices. All prices are subject to change without notice. POSTMASTER: Send address changes to *Obstetrics and Gynecology Clinics*, Elsevier Health Sciences Division, Subscription Customer Service, 3251 Riverport Lane, Maryland Heights, MO 63043. **Customer Service: Telephone: 1-800-654-2452 (U.S. and Canada); 314-447-8871 (outside U.S. and Canada). Fax: 314-447-8029. E-mail: journalscustomerservice-usa@elsevier.com (for print support); journalsonlinesupport-usa@elsevier. com (for online support).**

Reprints. For copies of 100 or more of articles in this publication, please contact the Commercial Reprints Department, Elsevier Inc., 360 Park Avenue South, New York, New York 10010-1710. Tel.: 212-633-3874; Fax: 212-633-3820; E-mail: reprints@elsevier.com.

Obstetrics and Gynecology Clinics of North America is also published in Spanish by McGraw-Hill Interamericana Editores S.A., P.O. Box 5-237, 06500, Mexico; in Portuguese by Reichmann and Affonso Editores, Rio de Janeiro, Brazil; and in Greek by Paschalidis Medical Publications, Athens, Greece.

Obstetrics and Gynecology Clinics of North America is covered in *MEDLINE/PubMed (Index Medicus), Excerpta Medica, Current Concepts/Clinical Medicine, Science Citation Index, BIOSIS, CINAHL, and ISI/BIOMED.*

Contributors

CONSULTING EDITOR

WILLIAM F. RAYBURN, MD, MBA
Affiliate Professor, Department of Obstetrics and Gynecology, College of Graduate
Studies, Medical University of South Carolina, Charleston, South Carolina; Emeritus
Distinguished Professor, Department of Obstetrics and Gynecology, University of New
Mexico School of Medicine, Albuquerque, New Mexico

EDITORS

KEVIN A. AULT, MD
Professor and Chair, Department of Obstetrics and Gynecology, Western Michigan
University Homer Stryker MD School of Medicine, Kalamazoo, Michigan

ALISA B. KACHIKIS, MD, MSc
Assistant Professor, Division of Maternal-Fetal Medicine, Department of Obstetrics and
Gynecology, University of Washington, Seattle, Washington

AUTHORS

ANNABETH BREWTON, MD
Department of Obstetrics and Gynecology, University of Tennessee Graduate School of
Medicine, Knoxville, Tennessee

DANA CANFIELD, MD
Maternal Fetal Medicine Fellow, Division of Maternal Fetal Medicine, Department of
Obstetrics, Gynecology and Reproductive Sciences, University of California, San Diego,
La Jolla, California

CATHERINE A. CHAPPELL, MD, MSc
Assistant Professor, Department of Obstetrics, Gynecology and Reproductive Sciences,
Magee-Womens Hospital and Magee-Womens Research Institute, Pittsburgh,
Pennsylvania

HYE CHO, BS
SUNY Upstate Medical University, Syracuse, New York

ANNIE M. DUDE, MD, PhD
Division of Maternal-Fetal Medicine, Department of Obstetrics and Gynecology, The
University of North Carolina at Chapel Hill, Chapel Hill, North Carolina

KARLEY DUTRA, MD
Clinical Instructor and Reproductive Infectious Disease Fellow, Department of Obstetrics and Gynecology, Medical University of South Carolina, Charleston, South Carolina

LINDA O. ECKERT, MD
Professor, Department of Obstetrics and Gynecology, Adjunct Department of Global Health, University of Washington School of Medicine, Seattle, Washington

SAMANTHA F. EHRLICH, PhD, MPH
Department of Public Health, University of Tennessee, Knoxville, Tennessee

SASCHA R. ELLINGTON, PhD
Division of Reproductive Health, National Center for Chronic Disease Prevention and Health Promotion, Centers for Disease Control and Prevention, Atlanta, Georgia

JANET A. ENGLUND, MD
Department of Pediatrics, Seattle Children's Hospital Pediatric Infectious Diseases, Seattle Children's Hospital Research Institute, University of Washington, Seattle, Washington

KATHERINE E. FLEMING-DUTRA, MD
National Center for Immunization and Respiratory Diseases, Centers for Disease Control and Prevention, Atlanta, Georgia

RACHEL S. FOGEL, BA
University of Pittsburgh School of Medicine, Pittsburgh, Pennsylvania

KIMBERLY B. FORTNER, MD
Department of Obstetrics and Gynecology, University of Tennessee Graduate School of Medicine, Knoxville, Tennessee

LAURYN GABBY, MD, FACOG
Maternal Fetal Medicine Fellow, Division of Maternal Fetal Medicine, Department of Obstetrics, Gynecology and Reproductive Sciences, University of California, San Diego, La Jolla, California

OLUWATOSIN GOJE, MD, MSCR
Associate Professor of Obstetrics, Gynecology and Reproductive Biology, Ob/Gyn and Women's Health Institute, Cleveland Clinic Foundation, Cleveland, Ohio

CYNTHIA GYAMFI-BANNERMAN, MD, MS, FACOG
Samuel SC Yen Endowed Chair, Division of Maternal Fetal Medicine, Department of Obstetrics, Gynecology and Reproductive Sciences, University of California, San Diego, La Jolla, California

MAUREEN S. HAMEL, MD
Assistant Professor, Department of Obstetrics and Gynecology, Providence, Rhode Island

FIONA HAVERS, MD
National Center for Immunization and Respiratory Diseases, Centers for Disease Control and Prevention, US Public Health Service Commissioned Corps, Atlanta, Georgia

DAVID M. HIGGINS, MD, MS
Department of Pediatrics, University of Colorado School of Medicine, Adult and Child Center for Health Outcomes Research and Delivery Science (ACCORDS), University of Colorado/Children's Hospital Colorado, Aurora, Colorado

TARA C. JATLAOUI, MD
US Public Health Service Commissioned Corps, Immunization Services Division, National Center for Immunization and Respiratory Diseases, Centers for Disease Control and Prevention, Atlanta, Georgia

MAURA JONES, MD
Division of Maternal-Fetal Medicine, Department of Obstetrics and Gynecology, The University of North Carolina at Chapel Hill, Chapel Hill, North Carolina

ALISA B. KACHIKIS, MD, MSc
Assistant Professor, Division of Maternal-Fetal Medicine, Department of Obstetrics and Gynecology, University of Washington, Seattle, Washington

GWENETH LAZENBY, MD, MSCP
Professor, Departments of Obstetrics and Gynecology and Internal Medicine, Medical University of South Carolina, Charleston, South Carolina

JILL M. MAPLES, PhD
Department of Obstetrics and Gynecology, University of Tennessee Graduate School of Medicine, Knoxville, Tennessee

JENNY Y. MEI, MD
Division of Maternal-Fetal Medicine, Department of Obstetrics and Gynecology, David Geffen School of Medicine at UCLA, Los Angeles, California

SEAN T. O'LEARY, MD, MPH
Department of Pediatrics, University of Colorado School of Medicine, Adult and Child Center for Health Outcomes Research and Delivery Science (ACCORDS), University of Colorado/Children's Hospital Colorado, Aurora, Colorado

SARA E. OLIVER, MD
National Center for Immunization and Respiratory Diseases, Centers for Disease Control and Prevention, US Public Health Service Commissioned Corps, Atlanta, Georgia

CHRISTINE K. OLSON, MD
Division of Healthcare Quality Promotion, National Center for Emerging and Zoonotic Infectious Diseases, Centers for Disease Control and Prevention, US Public Health Service Commissioned Corps, Atlanta, Georgia

KELSEY PETRIE, MD, MPH
Complex Family Planning Fellow, Department of Obstetrics and Gynecology, University of Washington School of Medicine, Seattle, Washington

ANNA MAYA POWELL, MD, MSc
Assistant Professor of Gynecology and Obstetrics, Johns Hopkins School of Medicine, Baltimore, Maryland

LAUREN E. ROPER, MPH
National Center for Immunization and Respiratory Diseases, Centers for Disease Control and Prevention, Atlanta, Georgia

ISABELLA SARRIA, BA
Johns Hopkins Bloomberg School of Public Health, Baltimore, Maryland

ANDREA J. SHARMA, PhD
Division of Healthcare Quality Promotion, National Center for Emerging and Zoonotic Infectious Diseases, Centers for Disease Control and Prevention, US Public Health Service Commissioned Corps, Atlanta, Georgia

NEIL S. SILVERMAN, MD
Division of Maternal-Fetal Medicine, Department of Obstetrics and Gynecology, David Geffen School of Medicine at UCLA, Los Angeles, California

BENJAMIN SPIRES, MD, Major, USAF, MC
Department of Obstetrics and Gynecology, Uniformed Services University of the Health Sciences, Eglin Air Force Base, Florida

NAOMI TEPPER, MD
US Public Health Service Commissioned Corps, Division of Birth Defects and Infant Disorders, National Center on Birth Defects and Developmental Disabilities, Centers for Disease Control and Prevention, Atlanta, Georgia

METHODIUS TUULI, MD, MPH, MBA
Professor and Chair, Department of Obstetrics and Gynecology, Providence, Rhode Island

EVELYN TWENTYMAN, MD
National Center for Immunization and Respiratory Diseases, Centers for Disease Control and Prevention, Atlanta, Georgia

ELMIRA VAZIRI FARD, MD, MPH
Gynecology Pathology Fellow, Department of Pathology and Lab Medicine, University of California, San Diego, La Jolla, California

ALEX WELLS, MD, MBs
Complex Family Planning Fellow, Department of Obstetrics and Gynecology, University of Washington School of Medicine, Seattle, Washington

TENISHA WILSON, MD, PhD
Division of Maternal-Fetal Medicine, Department of Obstetrics and Gynecology, The University of North Carolina at Chapel Hill, Chapel Hill, North Carolina

KATE R. WOODWORTH, MD
Division of Birth Defects and Infant Disorders, National Center on Birth Defects and Developmental Disabilities, Centers for Disease Control and Prevention, Atlanta, Georgia

LAUREN HEAD ZAUCHE, PhD, MSN
Division of Healthcare Quality Promotion, National Center for Emerging and Zoonotic Infectious Diseases, Centers for Disease Control and Prevention, Atlanta, Georgia

Contents

sensitive and specific test. Treatment with doxycycline or ceftriaxone is recommended for chlamydia and gonorrhea, respectively. Expedited partner therapy is cost-effective and acceptable by patients as a means to reduce transmission. Test of cure is indicated in persons at risk for reinfection or during pregnancy. Future directions include identifying effective strategies for prevention.

Vulvovaginitis occurs in mostly reproductive aged women. Recurrent vaginitis affects overall quality of life, with a large financial burden on the patient, family, and health system. This review discusses a clinician's approach to vulvovaginitis with specific attention to the 2021 updated Center for Disease Control and Prevention guidelines. The authors discuss the role of the microbiome in vaginitis and evidence-based approaches for diagnosis and treatment of vaginitis. This review also provides updates on new considerations, diagnosis, management, and treatment of vaginitis. Desquamative inflammatory vaginitis and genitourinary syndrome of menopause are discussed as differential diagnosis of vaginitis symptoms.

Cesarean delivery is the most common major surgical procedure performed among birthing persons in the United States, and surgical-site infection is a significant complication. Several significant advances in preventive measures have been shown to reduce infection risk, while others remain plausible but not yet proven in clinical trials.

Cervical cancer is the fourth most common cancer in women worldwide with immense associated morbidity and mortality. Although most of the cervical cancer cases are caused by the human papillomavirus (HPV) and can effectively be prevented by HPV vaccination, vaccination unfortunately remains underused on a global scale with vast inequities in distribution. A vaccine as a tool to prevent cancer, cervical and others, is largely unprecedented. Then why do HPV vaccination rates globally remain so low? This article explores the burden of disease, development of the vaccine and its subsequent uptake, cost-effectiveness, and associated equity issues.

Hepatitis B virus (HBV) is efficiently transmitted to newborn infants in the perinatal period and can lead to chronic infection, cirrhosis, liver cancer, and death. Despite the availability of effective prevention measures necessary to eliminate perinatal HBV transmission, significant gaps remain in the implementation of these prevention measures. All clinicians who care for pregnant persons and their newborn infants need to know the key prevention measures including (1) identification of HBV surface antigen (HBsAg)-positive pregnant persons, (2) antiviral treatment of HBsAg-positive pregnant persons with high viral loads, (3) timely postexposure prophylaxis of infants born to HBsAg-positive persons, (4) and timely universal vaccination of newborn infants.

With the advent of safe and well-tolerated direct-acting antiviral (DAA) medications for hepatitis C virus (HCV), disease eradication is on the horizon. However, as the rate of HCV infection among women of childbearing potential continues to rise due to the ongoing opioid epidemic in the United States, perinatal transmission of HCV presents an increasingly difficult barrier. Without the ability to treat HCV during pregnancy, complete eradication is unlikely. In this review, we discuss the current epidemiology of HCV in the United States, the current management strategy for HCV in pregnancy, as well as the potential for future use of DAAs in pregnancy.

To decrease risk of early-onset neonatal sepsis from group B streptococcus (GBS), pregnant patients should undergo screening between 36 0/7 and 37 6/7 weeks' gestation. Patients with a positive vaginal-rectal culture, GBS bacteriuria , or history of newborn with GBS disease should receive intrapartum antibiotic prophylaxis (IAP) with an agent targeting GBS. If GBS status is unknown at time of labor, IAP should be administered in cases of preterm birth, rupture of membranes for >18 hours, or intrapartum fever. The antibiotic of choice is intravenous penicillin; alternatives should be considered in cases of penicillin allergy depending on allergy severity.

Approximately 5000 people living with human immunodeficiency virus (HIV) give birth each year. Perinatal transmission of HIV will occur in about 15% to 45% of pregnancies without treatment. With appropriate antiretroviral therapy for pregnant people as well as appropriate intrapartum and postpartum interventions, the rate of perinatal transmission can be reduced to less than 1%. Antiretroviral therapy will also reduce health risks for pregnant patients living with HIV. All pregnant people should be offered the opportunity to learn their HIV status and access treatment as needed.

The development of vaccines is considered one of the greatest breakthroughs of modern medicine, saving millions of lives around the world each year. Despite vaccines' proven success, vaccine hesitancy remains a major issue affecting vaccine uptake. Common themes exist in patients' apprehension to receiving vaccines. Women's health providers possess an important role in addressing these concerns and dispelling common misconceptions that may increase vaccine hesitancy thereby reducing vaccine uptake. This review aims to explore many of these topics as they are related to women's health and provide strategies for providers to implement which may reduce vaccine hesitancy among our patients.

Alisa B. Kachikis, Hye Cho, and Janet A. Englund

Respiratory syncytial virus (RSV) infection is a significant cause of morbidity and mortality among infants aged younger than 1 year, adults aged 65 years or older, and immunocompromised persons. Limited data exist on RSV infection in pregnancy and further research is needed. Strides are being made to develop vaccines, including vaccines for maternal immunization, as well as monoclonal antibodies for disease prevention.

OBSTETRICS AND GYNECOLOGY CLINICS

SERIES OF RELATED INTEREST

Clinics in Perinatology
www.perinatology.theclinics.com
Pediatric Clinics of North America
https://www.pediatrics.theclinics.com

THE CLINICS ARE AVAILABLE ONLINE!
Access your subscription at:
www.theclinics.com

Foreword

Combating Growth of New and Old Infectious Diseases

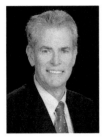

William F. Rayburn, MD, MBA
Consulting Editor

While a resident in training, I had the opportunity of working with a faculty member who returned after infectious disease fellowship training at the Centers for Disease Control and Prevention (CDC). Since that time, I have found that a faculty member with expertise in infectious disease is invaluable to our patient care and my education. It is a pleasure to welcome Kevin Ault, MD and Alisa Kachikis, MD as editors of this issue of *Obstetrics and Gynecology Clinics of North America* that deals with infectious diseases in obstetrics and gynecology. Both have organized an important issue dealing with topics of active interest to all women's health practitioners.

Since our last issue on this subject in 2014, we have become better informed about certain constantly changing and evolving infectious diseases. Not only did the COVID-19 pandemic thrust scrutiny on infectious disease epidemiology and prevention measures, but also the many sources of publicly available information required validation or limited interpretation. Health equity and maternal morbidity and mortality from infection have also gained considerable attention in recent years. Certain well-recognized infections, such as sexually transmitted infections (gonorrhea, chlamydia, and syphilis), are on the rise. Reviews of viral infections, such as cytomegalovirus, hepatitis B and C, HIV, and HPV, and different causes of vulvovaginitis remain relevant in relieving suffering and minimizing long-term consequences.

Highlighted in this issue are advances in research to improve treatment options in antibiotic regimens and to develop vaccines for use during pregnancy and in primary care. Despite these advancements, research initiatives in most clinical trials have not prioritized women's health due to either a lack of funding or exclusion of pregnant patients.

Vaccination and antimicrobial stewardship combat further drug use, adverse effects, and excess cost. A thorough history and physical examination are critical, particularly

Obstet Gynecol Clin N Am 50 (2023) xiii–xv
https://doi.org/10.1016/j.ogc.2023.03.015
0889-8545/23/© 2023 Published by Elsevier Inc.

obgyn.theclinics.com

for diagnostic dilemmas, such as a fever of unknown origin or presumed recurring or persistent infections. A sexual history, travel history, operative conditions, and recreational activities inform and help broaden the differential diagnosis. Rapid diagnostic testing, such as polymerase chain reaction (PCR), can provide early identification of an infectious agent or presence of antibiotic resistant genes (eg, medA gene).

Half of this issue pertains to pregnancy. Infections involve not only the reproductive tract organs of all women but also any organ system during pregnancy. There are no class A antimicrobials. Penicillin and cephalosporins (class B) are frequently used, while tetracyclines and fluoroquinolones are contraindicated. Sulfonamides and aminoglycosides should not be used if alternative agents are available. Many antimicrobials are eliminated in breast milk and should be used with caution, but not necessarily avoided, in breast-feeding women.

Empiric antimicrobial therapy is often used immediately against the most likely infecting organism(s). Knowing about any drug allergies, potential drug-drug interactions, microbiologic culture results, and prior antibiotic exposure helps guide more targeted drug selection. Renal and hepatic function testing are seldom necessary but can guide antimicrobial dosing regimens and any need for serum drug monitoring.

When treatment failure is suspected, we are trained to ask several questions: is the presumed organism the etiologic agent or a superinfection? Is the antimicrobial regimen appropriate and taken properly? Are adequate concentrations of the antimicrobial achieved at the site of infection? And, has source control been adequately accomplished? Another fundamental question is whether the shortest duration of therapy was identified for eradicating the infection. Generally speaking, treatment of an acute uncomplicated infection should be until the patient is afebrile and clinically well. A minimum of 72 hours is necessary unless there needs to be more prolonged therapy for infections outside the reproductive organs (eg, endocarditis, osteomyelitis, septic arthritis).

Half of this issue deals with benefits and hesitancies about vaccinations (eg, COVID-19, HPV, HIV, hepatitis B) that are particularly relevant to the obstetrician-gynecologist. I especially enjoyed reading the article pertaining to vaccine hesitancy in women's health and understanding roles of the patient's provider and family. The American College of Obstetricians and Gynecologists stresses the importance of integrating an effective vaccine strategy into the care of both obstetric and gynecologic patients. The College further emphasizes that information on the safety of vaccines given during pregnancy is subject to change, and recommendations can be found on the CDC Web site at www.cdc.gov/vaccines.

The women's health community must adapt to the changing times and treatment improvements of current and emerging pathogens. The clarity of these articles prepared by the experienced authors, with edits from Dr Ault and Dr Kachikis, directs our attention to combating new and old infectious diseases. We are indebted to this stellar group of authors for their cutting-edge contributions. Knowledge gleaned by the readers will assist in addressing some of the most important interventions, which are either evidence-based or emerging.

William F. Rayburn, MD, MBA
Department of Obstetrics and Gynecology
Medical University of South Carolina
1721 Atlantic Avenue
Sullivan's Island, SC 29482, USA

E-mail address:
wrayburnmd@gmail.com

Preface

Infectious Diseases in Obstetrics and Gynecology: Moving Forward in the Twenty-First Century

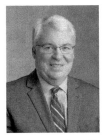 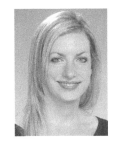

Kevin A. Ault, MD   Alisa B. Kachikis, MD, MSc
Editors

Infectious diseases are more important than ever in the twenty-first century. Not only did the COVID-19 pandemic catapult scrutiny of infectious disease epidemiology and prevention measures into the mainstream media and dinner table discussion, but also, thanks to social media, there are countless official and unofficial sources of information for public consumption. Emerging diseases continue to grab headlines, from COVID-19 to Mpox (or Monkeypox), Ebola virus and Marburg virus outbreaks and the "triple-demic" of COVID-19, influenza, and respiratory syncytial virus surges in 2022.

At the same time, maternal mortality and health equity measures require attention both nationally and globally. Infectious diseases contribute significantly to maternal morbidity and mortality, including surgical site infections and group B streptococcus sepsis. In addition, age-old infections, such as sexually transmitted infections, which were on the rise prior to the COVID-19 pandemic, are markedly increasing. Other infections such as cytomegalovirus, hepatitis B and hepatitis C viruses, HIV, and different causes for vaginitis, remain clinically important, causing suffering and often long-term consequences.

New technology and advances in research are contributing to improved prevention and treatment options in obstetrics and gynecology from changes in antibiotic regimens to development of vaccines for use in pregnancy and in primary care. The human papillomavirus (HPV) vaccine, for example, has enormous potential to decrease rates of cervical and other HPV-associated cancers. Despite these strides, it is glaringly apparent that women's health and research initiatives have been neglected over the decades in terms of funding and inclusion of reproductive age and pregnant individuals

Obstet Gynecol Clin N Am 50 (2023) xvii–xviii
https://doi.org/10.1016/j.ogc.2023.02.001
0889-8545/23/© 2023 Elsevier Inc. All rights reserved.

obgyn.theclinics.com

in clinical trials. In addition, inequities in distribution of these new technologies and vaccines are persistently present.

Over the last three years, it has been critical for obstetrics and gynecology care providers to become educated in constantly changing and evolving infectious disease topics to provide the best counseling, recommendations, and treatments for their patients. Research advances have led to potential vaccines and treatments on the horizon. The obstetrics and gynecology community—from professional organizations to academic centers and private practices to the prenatal or primary care providers—must remain agile to adapt to changing times and improve treatment for current infectious diseases impacting obstetrics and gynecology while also responding to emerging pathogens.

Kevin A. Ault, MD
Department of Obstetrics and Gynecology
Western Michigan University
Homer Stryker MD School of Medicine
1000 Oakland Drive
Kalamazoo, MI 49008, USA

Alisa B. Kachikis, MD, MSc
Division of Maternal-Fetal Medicine
Department of Obstetrics & Gynecology
University of Washington
1959 NE Pacific Street
Box 356460
Seattle, WA 98195, USA

E-mail addresses:
kevin.ault@med.wmich.edu (K.A. Ault)
abk26@uw.edu (A.B. Kachikis)

Cytomegalovirus in Pregnancy

Dana Canfield, MD[a,1], Lauryn Gabby, MD, FACOG[a,1], Elmira Vaziri Fard, MD, MPH[b,2], Cynthia Gyamfi-Bannerman, MD, MS, FACOG[a,*]

KEYWORDS

- Cytomegalovirus in pregnancy • Screening for congenital cytomegalovirus
- Ultrasonographic findings

KEY POINTS

- Cytomegalovirus (CMV) is a common maternal infection that contributes significantly to neonatal morbidity and mortality.
- Detection of congenital CMV in the prenatal period is reasonably accurate due to several sonographic markers and a high diagnostic accuracy using polymerase chain reaction of amniotic fluid.
- There are currently no proven strategies for prenatal prevention or antenatal treatment.

INTRODUCTION AND BACKGROUND
Significance and Prevalence

Cytomegalovirus (CMV) is a common double-stranded DNA herpesvirus. Due both to the prevalence of the virus and the potential severity of its sequelae, CMV remains a major cause of neonatal morbidity and mortality. The leading nongenetic cause of neonatal deafness, congenital CMV occurs in roughly 0.6% to 0.7% of all live births in high-income countries[1] and disproportionately burdens individuals in low-resource settings globally.[2] CMV is also an expensive disease with the annual costs associated with treating resulting disabilities and complications totaling more than US$1.86 billion annually.[3]

TRANSMISSION, PREVENTION, AND RISK FACTORS
Transmission

The threat that congenital CMV poses to international health is underscored by its disease course and transmission. In the United States, roughly 50% of adults will be

[a] Division of Maternal Fetal Medicine, Department of Obstetrics, Gynecology & Reproductive Sciences, University of California, San Diego, CA, USA; [b] Department of Pathology and Lab Medicine, University of California, San Diego, CA, USA
[1] Present address: 9300 Campus Point Drive, MC 7433, La Jolla, California 92037, USA.
[2] Present address: 9444 Medical Center Drive, Suite I-027, La Jolla, CA 92037, USA.
* Corresponding author. 9300 Campus Point Drive, MC 7433, La Jolla, CA 92037-1300.
E-mail address: cgyamfibannerman@health.ucsd.edu

Obstet Gynecol Clin N Am 50 (2023) 263–277
https://doi.org/10.1016/j.ogc.2023.02.002
0889-8545/23/© 2023 Elsevier Inc. All rights reserved.
obgyn.theclinics.com

seropositive by age of 40 years,[4] and among children and immunocompetent adults, infection is generally asymptomatic.[5] For those who do have symptoms, they are usually mild and vague, consisting of malaise, low-grade fevers, aches, and lymphadenopathy.[3] Given the prevalence and indolent course of the infection, most adults worldwide have been infected by CMV at some point but remain unaware, contributing to its spread and impact.

Further, such as other viruses in the herpesvirus family, CMV can remain latent in the host cells following an initial infection and has the potential to become reactivated and transmitted.[5] The highest concentrations of CMV are found in the plasma, urine, seminal fluid, saliva, and breast milk of individuals that have been recently infected.[5]

Thus, horizontal transmission generally occurs through close contact between individuals but rarely occurs through blood transfusion or organ transplant.[4] Vertical transmission can also occur in several ways, most commonly through transplacental infection, during delivery, or through breastfeeding.[4]

Because of its widespread prevalence and multiple routes of transmission, pregnant individuals frequently encounter CMV. Among women of childbearing age, 30% to 50% are susceptible to primary infection and 50% to 70% are susceptible to secondary infection.[6] Among previously seronegative pregnant individuals, the incidence of primary maternal CMV infection is approximately 0.7% to 4%, whereas the incidence of secondary infection is reportedly as high as 13%.[7–9] The risk of transmission to the fetus greatly depends on whether it results from a primary infection in pregnancy or a secondary infection. In the case of a primary infection, 30% to 50% of neonates will become infected compared with only 0.5% to 2% with mothers who were previously seropositive[10–13] (Fig. 1). Infants who contract CMV because of a primary maternal infection are also more likely to have severe sequelae.[5,14]

Maternal viremia can lead to placental infection with preferential infection of the pericyte cells, as demonstrated by placental histopathology examination.[15] However, not all fetuses become infected. Although the mechanism is unknown, the placenta may play a major protective role in preventing vertical transmission. This is most easily demonstrated in discordant twin pairs, where one twin becomes infected with CMV and the other does not.[16–19] Researchers studying these twin pairs further concluded that the placental type in multifetal gestations does not predict the pattern of vertical transmission or the clinical course after delivery.[19,20] Limited reports have also suggested that prenatal horizontal infection is possible given positive CMV polymerase chain reaction (PCR) of the amniotic fluid of only one twin with both infants testing positive after delivery and placental findings to strongly suggest transmission between twins.[19,21]

Risk Factors for Transmission

Given its spread through saliva and urine, individuals who perform childcare duties are at the highest risk of contracting CMV.[13] An estimated 50% of children in daycare shed CMV leaving daycare workers, parents, and teachers highly susceptible to infection. This is particularly true in the setting of other risk factors such as immunocompromise and chronic illness.[22] Surprisingly, seronegative health-care workers, including those working in a pediatric setting, are not at an increased risk.[23] A variety of socioeconomic factors have been studied in connection with CMV infection. Some, such as education level, have been linked to increased rates of seropositivity, whereas others, such as income and race, are not consistently linked.[2]

Pregnant individuals face unique considerations related to risk of vertical transmission and congenital infection. As previously mentioned, primary infection in pregnancy is much more likely to result both in transmission to a fetus and severe sequelae.

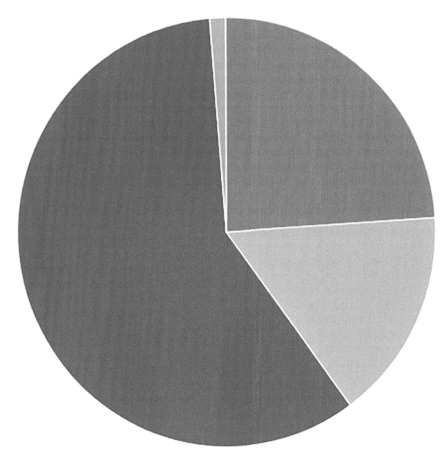

- Individuals Susceptible to Primary Infection in Pregnancy   • Rate of Vertical Transmission following Primary Infection
- Individuals Susceptible to Secondary Infection in Pregnancy   • Rate of Vertical Transmission following Secondary Infection

Fig. 1. CMV status and risk of transmission in pregnancy.

Further, timing of infection during pregnancy plays a major role in the risk of transmission and of severe sequelae; infants whose mothers were infected in the third trimester are at the highest risk of infection, with reports of transmission as high as 50%.[5] However, the likelihood of severe morbidity is by far the highest in the first trimester, particularly in the setting of primary infection; in these circumstances, about 5% to 15% of infants will be symptomatic at birth.[5] In summary, when it comes to avoiding vertical transmission, there is no "safe" time for a pregnant individual to be exposed to CMV.

Prevention

Although public interest in CMV has led to the study of several strategies at various phases of the infectious course, there is currently no antenatal treatment or prenatal prevention strategy aside from behavioral modifications. Three approaches, including immunoglobulin treatment, antiviral therapy, and vaccination, will be discussed below and are summarized in **Box 1**.

Administration of hyperimmune globulin to women with primary CMV infection in pregnancy garnered significant attention when several small observational studies demonstrated a potential reduction in the incidence of vertical transmission.[12] The small size and inconclusive results of these studies prompted a larger, definitive randomized trial conducted from 2012 to 2018.[24] This trial included 712 pregnant participants with singleton fetuses who were less than 23 weeks gestation and were found to have a primary CMV infection based on either elevated IgM and IgG antibody levels with IgG avidity less than 50% or a positive IgG after a negative IgG screen earlier in pregnancy. These patients were randomized to either received CMV hyperimmune globulin or placebo in monthly infusions until delivery, and the primary outcome was confirmed fetal infection or congenital infection diagnosed by 3 weeks of age or neonatal death without CMV testing. Ultimately, there was no benefit to treatment with CMV hyperimmune globulin with a primary outcome rate of 22.7% of the hyperimmune globulin group and 19.4% of the placebo group. The trial was stopped early due to futility.[24]

Antiviral therapies have also been tested in several small studies.[25,26] One study published in 2021 screened patients via serology before 14 weeks and offered those with positive serology treatment with high-dose valacyclovir with amniocentesis performed at 17 to 22 weeks gestation to assess for fetal infection via PCR. A total of 65 patients were treated, and fetal infection was significantly lower in the treated group (odds ratio 0.318 [95% confidence interval, 0.120–0.841]; $P = 0.021$).[27] Another similar randomized controlled trial in 2020 of 100 patients demonstrated similarly promising results for women who acquired CMV periconceptionally or in the first trimester and were treated with high-dose valacyclovir.[28] Although the limited data are promising, a larger randomized controlled trial is needed to further validate this approach before considering widespread implementation. In addition, this strategy would require universal screening in pregnancy, which is currently not performed for several reasons to be discussed in the next section of this review.

Another investigated strategy prevention of CMV transmission is through vaccination. Attempts at CMV vaccine development with the specific aim of preventing congenital CMV have been ongoing since the 1970s,[29] thwarted by several factors. First, for many years, there was a lack of awareness of the threat posed by congenital CMV that lead to stagnant research efforts given a paucity of interest in prevention of

---

Box 1
Preventative strategies for cytomegalovirus

Suggested Preventative Strategies for CMV transmission
- *Frequent handwashing* or *use of gloves* after the following activities:
  - Diaper changes
  - Feeding and meal preparation/cleanup
  - Wiping a child's nose
  - Handling bottles, pacifiers, sippy cups, and other utensils

- *Avoid the following activities* while performing childcare:
  - Sharing utensils, food, and beverages
  - Kissing

Previously Studied Preventative Strategies
- Hyperimmune globulin
  - Efficacy disproven in a large, definitive RCT

- Antivirals
  - Potential efficacy based on limited data; large RCT needed

- Vaccines
  - Several under development; Phase 3 Trial needed

the virus and funding for the development of a vaccine. Second, there are several immunogenic properties of the virus that make vaccine development challenging, including its ability to evade the immune system.[29] Although multiple vaccines have advanced to the Phase II trial stage of development, creating a vaccine that is durable without toxicity has been a challenge for researchers.[29] Although there is not currently a vaccine available, there are several in development aimed specifically at the prevention of congenital CMV.[30]

Although further investigation into novel methods continues, hygiene-based behavioral modifications remain the mainstay of prevention (see **Box 1**). A prospective study of 5312 seronegative pregnant patients recruited at 12 weeks gestation demonstrated a lower than expected rate of seroconversion when tested again at 36 weeks.[31] A 2020 systematic review of 7 studies implementing educational interventions concluded that the nonrandomized design and heterogeneity of these studies preclude a conclusion regarding their utility.[32] Although a larger, randomized study would be necessary to prove the efficacy of educational interventions, the available evidence supports the low risk of harm and simplicity of educational interventions.[23]

OBSERVATION/ASSESSMENT/EVALUATION
Universal Serologic Screening is Not Recommended

There are several important considerations related to CMV screening during prenatal care. First, universal screening is not recommended by American College of Obstetricians and Gynecologists (ACOG) or Society for Maternal-Fetal Medicine (SMFM).[3,6] Epidemiologic principles of screening state that there should be a readily available and acceptable treatment and an accurate screening test to screen for a condition.[33] As discussed in the last section, although several therapies aimed at preventing transmission have been studied, none has demonstrated acceptable efficacy for routine use.

As we will later discuss, when congenital CMV has been diagnosed, there are no proven treatment options (**Fig. 2**). Accuracy of screening poses a further issue, particularly in the absence of findings that make the diagnosis more likely. It is difficult to determine whether maternal IgM antibodies are the result of a primary versus recurrent infection because these antibodies can remain in maternal circulation for months following infection.[34] For the same reason, it is not possible to know whether infection was present at the time of organogenesis based on serology screening.[35] Counseling patients who screen positive regarding fetal risks is therefore quite difficult.

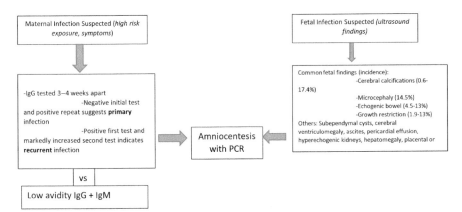

Fig. 2. Recommended pathways to diagnosing congenital CMV.

Appropriate Patients for Maternal Serologic Screening

Although universal screening is discouraged, there are some scenarios in which it is appropriate to send serologic studies with the aim of detecting a maternal CMV infection. These mainly consist of cases in which exposure to CMV during pregnancy is strongly suspected based on exposure to individuals known to be infected, or in the case of maternal symptoms in the setting of immunosuppression. As both children and immunocompetent adults are commonly asymptomatic, it is unusual that a patient presenting to for prenatal care is identified for CMV screening based on symptoms or a potential exposure.[5]

Immunosuppressed individuals are the exception and can have a very serious disease with clinical manifestations consisting of CMV retinitis, hepatitis, pneumonitis, and gastrointestinal distress.[36] Given limited evidence to guide the care of immunocompromised pregnant patients and the potential severity of infectious sequelae in these patients, a multidisciplinary approach should be utilized when managing these patients. With increasing numbers of pregnancies complicated with conditions such as lupus, solid organ transplant, and human immunodeficiency virus (HIV), it is important to maintain a low threshold for screening when providing prenatal care for these patients if they develop concerning symptoms. Because antiviral treatments are used in their nonpregnant counterparts to prevent tissue damage in select cases, there may be a role for their use in immunocompromised pregnant patients in the right clinical setting.

When maternal CMV is clinically suspected, repeat anti-CMV IgG titers should be sent 3 to 4 weeks after the initial testing. Seroconversion during this time period suggests a primary infection and a significant (eg, 4-fold) increase in titers suggests recurrent infection.[3] Alternatively, IgG avidity testing can help detect newer IgG antibodies if available; the combination of a positive IgM positive IgG with low avidity is approximately 92% sensitive for detecting a recent maternal CMV infection.[3,6]

Suspected Fetal Infection

When serologies diagnose a primary maternal CMV infection or a reinfection, a detailed anatomic fetal ultrasound examination should be performed, and the patient should be offered an amniocentesis with amniotic fluid sent for PCR.[6] Previous studies have examined cordocentesis as a method for detection but when weighing the procedural risks against diagnostic accuracy amniocentesis has become the sampling method of choice.[3,6,37] A diagnosis can be confirmed by PCR for CMV DNA and viral load on amniotic fluid. To give the most accurate results, amniocentesis should be done at greater than 21 weeks gestation and at least 6 weeks from the suspected maternal infection.[6] In this setting, amniocentesis has a specificity of 97% to 100%.[38–40] A high viral load defined as greater than 100,000 copies/mL was discovered to be a strong predictor of adverse perinatal outcomes in one retrospective multicenter study.[41]

In possible discordantly infected twin gestations, Lazzarotto and colleagues[21] suggest amniocentesis with PCR be performed after 21 weeks gestation and at least 6 to 8 weeks after suspected maternal infection, similar to singleton gestations.

Ultrasound Findings

Due to the high frequency of asymptomatic CMV infections, congenital CMV is more frequently suspected based on abnormal ultrasound findings. However, it should be noted that when[42] fetal infection status is unknown, ultrasound abnormalities predict symptomatic congenital infection in only a third of cases. The most frequent ultrasound findings include echogenic bowel (4.5%–13% of fetuses; **Fig. 3**); CNS findings, which include ventriculomegaly (**Fig. 4**C), cerebral calcifications, subependymal

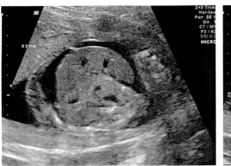
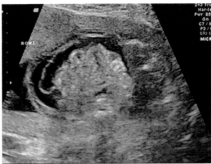

Fig. 3. Ascites and echogenic bowel on a fetus with congenital CMV.

cysts, and microcephaly (4.5%–17.4% of fetuses; **Fig. 4**A and B); and fetal growth restriction (1.9%–13% of fetuses).[6] Other relatively common findings include hydrops and its separate components (ascites, pericardial effusion, and placentamegaly), hyperechogenic kidneys, hepatomegaly (**Fig. 5**), and hepatic calcifications.[6] Given that these findings are all found as a result of several other causes, including many genetic disorders, the authors of one study sought to find a unique marker and discovered that an anechoic cavity located on the extremity of the occipital horn was frequently noted in fetuses with confirmed CMV both by amniotic fluid PCR and after birth by urine analysis in liveborn babies.[43] More studies are needed to corroborate this finding.

The question of whether to use MRI to enhance the sensitivity of imaging to detect congenital CMV has been considered. In general, it remains controversial with limited data to support its use,[37] leading SMFM to recommend against using it routinely.[6]

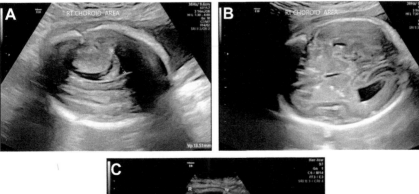
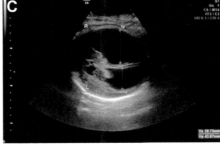

Fig. 4. (A–C) Cerebral calcification and ventriculomegaly seen on a fetus with congenital CMV.

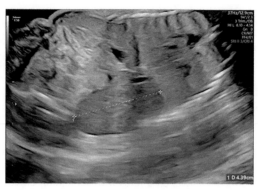

Fig. 5. Hepatomegaly in a fetus with congenital CMV.

Limitations of Ultrasound

It is worth noting that ultrasound has limited sensitivity in detecting congenital CMV but that affected fetuses without sonographic findings are less likely to have severe sequelae. The authors of a 2008 study reviewing sonographic images of neonates that were found to be symptomatic with CMV concluded that when fetal infection status is unknown, ultrasound abnormalities predict symptomatic congenital infection in only a third of cases.[44] A 2021 meta-analysis of studies including fetuses diagnosed with congenital CMV without ultrasound findings concluded that 45.3% of 2603 fetuses studied had ultrasound findings. However, the authors reported rates of adverse developmental outcomes in 1% to 6% of infants without ultrasound findings compared with 15% to 25% in infants with prenatal ultrasound findings consistent with CMV.[42]

ANTENATAL TREATMENT/MONITORING

Data on efficacious treatment options of CMV in pregnancy is limited, and unfortunately, there are currently no recommended antepartum therapies for documented maternal or fetal infection. As previously mentioned, hyperimmune globulins initially showed promise as a method for preventing vertical transmission of CMV in the case of primary maternal infection and in reducing sequelae[12,45] but the effectiveness of this therapy was later disproven by a definitive randomized trial.[24]

Valacyclovir, as briefly discussed earlier, has been suggested as a potential treatment option. It is classified as pregnancy group B, which denotes no clear evidence of human risk when taken during pregnancy; however, there is a paucity of data regarding its efficacy. The use of valacyclovir for symptomatic congenital CMV infection was first reported by Jacquemard and colleagues in 2007.[46] Twenty-one cases of PCR-confirmed fetal CMV were included. Cordocentesis was performed to examine platelet count and liver function as surrogate markers for symptomatic fetal infection. High-dose treatment of 2 g 4 times per day was initiated at a median of 28 weeks and continued for 7 weeks. Although CMV viral load decreased, there was no difference in the rates of neonatal morbidity and mortality compared with a CMV positive cohort that was not treated. Additionally, their findings were not stratified further by severity of fetal infection. This same group later completed a prospective cohort study of 41 confirmed fetal CMV cases.[47] In cases where infection was confirmed by amniocenteses, valacyclovir 8 g per day was administered. Severely affected fetuses, defined as those with cerebral calcifications, and asymptomatic fetuses were excluded. In the moderately affected group, viral loads decreased by a mean of $-0.5 \log_{10}$IU/mL

($P = .01$) and fetal platelet count increased by a mean of 101,000 ($P < .001$) between the initiation of treatment and birth. This group compared their findings to historical controls and determined that valacyclovir treatment increased the frequency of asymptomatic neonates from 43% to 82% with treatment.

A separate randomized controlled trial evaluated the use of valacyclovir 500 mg twice daily for its effect on HIV viral load suppression in herpes simplex virus-2-affected patients.[28] However, the authors also evaluated the effect on CMV. The authors concluded that there was a modest decrease in cervical shedding of CMV, although there was no effect on vertical transmission or breastmilk CMV viral loads. There are also select case reports on valacyclovir use for the prevention of vertical transmission, which demonstrated seronegative infants at birth and no maternal side effects of the medication.[48,49]

Currently, SMFM does not recommend treatment with valacyclovir, ganciclovir, or hyperimmune globulin. If antenatal therapy is considered, then it should only be offered in the context of a research protocol.[6]

Monitoring of Infected Fetuses

Given the high degree of variability among congenital CMV severity and its sequelae, there is limited guidance on the specifics of antenatal care for impacted patients. For patients with significant findings such as severe growth restriction and hydrops, careful planning for delivery between obstetric and neonatal teams should be undertaken with close monitoring leading up to delivery. However, even when maternal infection has been detected but there are no associated sonographic findings, regular monitoring for growth through ultrasounds and antenatal testing are still recommended given the increased risk developing severe findings that may alter management. Although neither ACOG nor SMFM give specific recommendations for surveillance, a reasonable strategy would be to perform repeat ultrasounds every 2 weeks after 24 weeks to monitor for hydrops or other signs of worsening fetal status and to initiate weekly or biweekly antenatal testing at 32 weeks.

Assessment after delivery

Following delivery, infants in whom CMV is suspected should be carefully evaluated for potential sequelae. The most common among these include low birthweight, head circumference below the 10th percentile, jaundice, petechiae, thrombocytopenia, and hepatosplenomegaly. In addition to providing immediate supportive care, pediatricians should also send a sample of urine or saliva for CMV PCR within 21 days of life to confirm the diagnosis.[50]

The placenta of any infant with suspected CMV should also be sent for PCR and histopathologic evaluation in order to provide further confirmation of infection or offer an alternative explanation for physical findings (eg, fetal growth restriction with findings related to placental insufficiency). On pathologic examination, the infected placenta is typically either large and pale or small and fibrotic. The most common histopathologic characteristics include villous fibrosis, villous stromal plasma cells infiltrate (**Fig. 6**), and characteristic large intranuclear inclusions with or without cytoplasmic inclusions (**Fig. 7**). If characteristic intranuclear inclusion cannot be identified on regular H&E examination, an immunohistochemical study can help to identify the cells that are infected by CMV2 (**Fig. 8**).

Neonatal Treatment

As in the case of treating maternal CMV infection in pregnancy, there is unfortunately no current evidence-based option for the treatment of the neonate. Supportive care

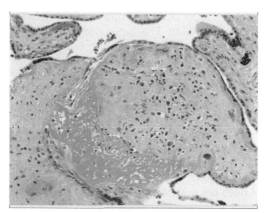

Fig. 6. Photomicrograph showing villous fibrosis and plasma cell infiltration (200×).

may include transfusion with blood products for patients with anemia or thrombocy-topenia.[50] Antivirals have been studied and show possible efficacy but data are currently limited.[50]

Breastfeeding Considerations

Patients should be counseled regarding the risks and benefits of breastfeeding in the setting of maternal CMV infection with a seronegative infant. Parents should be reassured that healthy, term neonates who breastfeed in these circumstances will generally remain asymptomatic,[51,52] and given the known benefits of breastfeeding, parents should consider this option. However, premature and very low birthweight babies may be at a greater risk of contracting infection, requiring a more in-depth discussion. One recent study indicated that half of preterm and very low birth weight infants exposed to CMV-positive breastmilk become infected, and a fifth develops severe clinical symptoms.[53] According to several studies, viral shedding can be detected in breastmilk from the time of delivery up to 9 months postpartum.[54] Severe symptoms described in this study were either sepsis or symptoms in at least 3 of the following categories: infection, bone marrow suppression, gastrointestinal or respiratory symptoms, and general appearance. Given the serious nature of these complications, particularly in an infant who is already compromised by prematurity or a low birthweight, the risk of

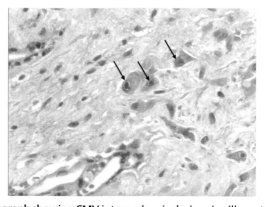

Fig. 7. Photomicrograph showing CMV intranuclear inclusions in villous stromal cells (400×).

Fig. 8. Immunohistochemical study for CMV highlights the infected cells (200×).

transmission should be seriously considered. If donor breastmilk is available to these infants, this may provide the nutritional benefits without the potential for infection.

NEONATAL FOLLOW-UP

One important aspect of the care of affected neonates concerns the delayed presentation of several commonly associated sequelae. Around 5% of infants who were asymptomatic at birth will go on to develop sequelae.[55] Although one study correlating viral load with sequelae discovered that neonates with a viral load of less than 3000 IU/dL rarely developed sensorineural deafness, there is no way to predict who among those with higher viral loads will develop deafness.[47] It is therefore important to regularly screen impacted infants for development of sensorineural hearing loss and cognitive conditions through early childhood because early detection allows for timely intervention and rehabilitation.[55] Although congenital hearing loss is usually the most severe symptom of secondary maternal infections,[22,56] mortality remains around 0.5% and 17% to 20% of surviving children have one or more long-term sequelae.

DISCUSSION/SUMMARY

CMV is a common, potentially morbid condition. Despite our ability to diagnose maternal CMV infection prenatally with reasonable accuracy, there are currently no well-studied methods to prevent fetal transmission or to treat neonates. Several strategies for the treatment and prevention have been studied, with immunoglobulins demonstrating a lack of efficacy in a large definitive trial, antivirals demonstrating potential efficacy in limited data, and the development of a vaccine underway for several decades with several factors hindering success. Hygienic practices bolstered by education provided by clinicians remain the cornerstone of prevention. Nonetheless, timely detection allows for improved screening for sequelae that require monitoring and intervention during both the prenatal and neonatal periods.

CLINICS CARE POINTS

- CMV infection in pregnancy is frequently asymptomatic. Serologic testing for CMV may be offered for individuals who develop influenza-like symptoms or if there are sonographic findings present.

- The diagnosis of primary CMV infection in pregnancy should be based on seroconversion in a previously seronegative individual, or the detection of IgM antibody with low IgG avidity.
- Secondary CMV infection is supported by a significant (eg, 4-fold) increase in IgG antibody titer with or without IgM and high avidity IgG.
- With primary maternal CMV infection, there is a 30% to 50% risk of transmission to the fetus.
- Prenatal diagnosis of fetal CMV infection is confirmed by PCR of viral DNA on amniotic fluid. Amniocentesis should be performed after 21 weeks gestation and after 6 to 8 weeks of suspected maternal infection.
- Fetal diagnosis and prognosis are not always concordant in multifetal gestations.
- In suspected and confirmed fetal CMV, cases should be followed with serial ultrasound examinations, which can track growth and examine for any developing anatomical findings that may aid in determining the prognosis for the neonate.
- Currently, there are no recommended treatment strategies for CMV infection in pregnancy.
- Breastfeeding is not absolutely contraindicated for mothers who develop primary CMV infection in pregnancy but should involve a discussion of risks and benefits, particularly for low birthweight or premature infants.

DISCLOSURE

None of the authors has funding from sources related to the topics covered in this review.

REFERENCES

1. Kenneson A, Cannon MJ. Review and meta-analysis of the epidemiology of congenital cytomegalovirus (CMV) infection. Rev Med Virol 2007;17(4):253–76.
2. Fowler K, Mucha J, Neumann M, et al. A systematic literature review of the global seroprevalence of cytomegalovirus: possible implications for treatment, screening, and vaccine development. BMC Public Health 2022;22(1):1659.
3. Practice bulletin no. 151: Cytomegalovirus, parvovirus B19, varicella zoster, and toxoplasmosis in pregnancy. Obstet Gynecol 2015;125(6):1510–25.
4. Clinical Overview. Centers for Disease Control and Prevention. 2022. Available at: https://www.cdc.gov/cmv/clinical/overview.html. Accessed Oct 17, 2022.
5. Resnik R, Lockwood CJ, Moore T, et al. Creasy and resnik's maternal-fetal medicine, 8th ed., 2018, Elsevier, Philadelphia, PA, 1, online resource (xviii, 1388 pages).
6. Hughes BL, Gyamfi-Bannerman C. (SMFM) SfM-FM. Diagnosis and antenatal management of congenital cytomegalovirus infection. Am J Obstet Gynecol 2016;214(6):B5–11.
7. Hagay ZJ, Biran G, Ornoy A, et al. Congenital cytomegalovirus infection: a long-standing problem still seeking a solution. Am J Obstet Gynecol 1996;174(1 Pt 1): 241–5.
8. Stagno S, Tinker MK, Elrod C, et al. Immunoglobulin M antibodies detected by enzyme-linked immunosorbent assay and radioimmunoassay in the diagnosis of cytomegalovirus infections in pregnant women and newborn infants. J Clin Microbiol 1985;21(6):930–5.
9. Colugnati FA, Staras SA, Dollard SC, et al. Incidence of cytomegalovirus infection among the general population and pregnant women in the United States. BMC Infect Dis 2007;7:71.

10. Revello MG, Lazzarotto T, Guerra B, et al. A randomized trial of hyperimmune globulin to prevent congenital cytomegalovirus. N Engl J Med 2014;370(14): 1316–26.

11. Stagno S, Pass RF, Cloud G, et al. Primary cytomegalovirus infection in pregnancy. Incidence, transmission to fetus, and clinical outcome. JAMA 1986; 256(14):1904–8.

12. Nigro G, Adler SP, La Torre R, et al. Passive immunization during pregnancy for congenital cytomegalovirus infection. N Engl J Med 2005;353(13):1350–62.

13. Fowler KB, Stagno S, Pass RF. Maternal immunity and prevention of congenital cytomegalovirus infection. JAMA 2003;289(8):1008–11.

14. Gabbe SG. Obstetrics : normal and problem pregnancies. 6th ed. Philadelphia, PA: Elsevier/Saunders; 2012. p. 1118–9.

15. Megli CJ, Coyne CB. Infections at the maternal-fetal interface: an overview of pathogenesis and defence. Nat Rev Microbiol 2022;20(2):67–82.

16. Carvalho AA, Silva CB, Martins ML, et al. Congenital cytomegalovirus infection in twin pregnancy. BMJ Case Rep 2021;14(7). https://doi.org/10.1136/bcr-2021-242712.

17. Egaña-Ugrinovic G, Goncé A, García L, et al. Congenital cytomegalovirus infection among twin pairs. J Matern Fetal Neonatal Med 2016;29(21):3439–44.

18. Ahlfors K, Ivarsson SA, Nilsson H. On the unpredictable development of congenital cytomegalovirus infection. A study in twins. Early Hum Dev 1988;18(2–3): 125–35.

19. Yinon Y, Yagel S, Tepperberg-Dikawa M, et al. Prenatal diagnosis and outcome of congenital cytomegalovirus infection in twin pregnancies. BJOG 2006;113(3): 295–300.

20. Saigal S, Eisele WA, Chernesky MA. Congenital cytomegalovirus infection in a pair of dizygotic twins. Am J Dis Child 1982;136(12):1094–5.

21. Lazzarotto T, Gabrielli L, Foschini MP, et al. Congenital cytomegalovirus infection in twin pregnancies: viral load in the amniotic fluid and pregnancy outcome. Pediatrics 2003;112(2):e153–7.

22. Fowler KB, Stagno S, Pass RF, et al. The outcome of congenital cytomegalovirus infection in relation to maternal antibody status. N Engl J Med 1992;326(10): 663–7.

23. Adler SP, Nigro G. Prevention of maternal-fetal transmission of cytomegalovirus. Clin Infect Dis 2013;57(Suppl 4):S189–92.

24. Hughes BL, Clifton RG, Rouse DJ, et al. A trial of hyperimmune globulin to prevent congenital cytomegalovirus infection. N Engl J Med 2021;385(5):436–44.

25. Zammarchi L, Lazzarotto T, Andreoni M, et al. Management of cytomegalovirus infection in pregnancy: is it time for valacyclovir? Clin Microbiol Infect 2020; 26(9):1151–4.

26. Marsico C, Kimberlin DW. Congenital Cytomegalovirus infection: advances and challenges in diagnosis, prevention and treatment. Ital J Pediatr 2017;43(1):38.

27. Faure-Bardon V, Fourgeaud J, Stirnemann J, et al. Secondary prevention of congenital cytomegalovirus infection with valacyclovir following maternal primary infection in early pregnancy. Ultrasound Obstet Gynecol 2021;58(4):576–81.

28. Shahar-Nissan K, Pardo J, Peled O, et al. Valaciclovir to prevent vertical transmission of cytomegalovirus after maternal primary infection during pregnancy: a randomised, double-blind, placebo-controlled trial. Lancet 2020;396(10253): 779–85.

29. Plotkin S. The history of vaccination against cytomegalovirus. Med Microbiol Immunol 2015;204(3):247–54.

30. Plotkin SA, Wang D, Oualim A, et al. The status of vaccine development against the human cytomegalovirus. J Infect Dis 2020;221(Suppl 1):S113–22.
31. Vauloup-Fellous C, Picone O, Cordier AG, et al. Does hygiene counseling have an impact on the rate of CMV primary infection during pregnancy? Results of a 3-year prospective study in a French hospital. J Clin Virol 2009;46(Suppl 4): S49–53.
32. Barber V, Calvert A, Vandrevala T, et al. Prevention of Acquisition of Cytomegalovirus Infection in Pregnancy Through Hygiene-based Behavioral Interventions: A Systematic Review and Gap Analysis. Pediatr Infect Dis J 2020;39(10):949–54.
33. Nielsen C, Lang RS. Principles of screening. Med Clin North Am 1999;83(6): 1323–37.
34. Lumley S, Patel M, Griffiths PD. The combination of specific IgM antibodies and IgG antibodies of low avidity does not always indicate primary infection with cytomegalovirus. J Med Virol 2014;86(5):834–7.
35. Ahmed B, Konje JC. Screening for infections in pregnancy - An overview of where we are today. Eur J Obstet Gynecol Reprod Biol 2021;263:85–93.
36. Dioverti MV, Razonable RR. Cytomegalovirus. Microbiol Spectr 2016;4(4). https:// doi.org/10.1128/microbiolspec.DMIH2-0022-2015.
37. Lazzarotto T, Guerra B, Lanari M, et al. New advances in the diagnosis of congenital cytomegalovirus infection. J Clin Virol 2008;41(3):192–7.
38. Enders G, Bäder U, Lindemann L, et al. Prenatal diagnosis of congenital cytomegalovirus infection in 189 pregnancies with known outcome. Prenat Diagn 2001;21(5):362–77.
39. Liesnard C, Donner C, Brancart F, et al. Prenatal diagnosis of congenital cytomegalovirus infection: prospective study of 237 pregnancies at risk. Obstet Gynecol 2000;95(6 Pt 1):881–8.
40. Donner C, Liesnard C, Brancart F, et al. Accuracy of amniotic fluid testing before 21 weeks' gestation in prenatal diagnosis of congenital cytomegalovirus infection. Prenat Diagn 1994;14(11):1055–9.
41. Mappa I, De Vito M, Flacco ME, et al. Prenatal predictors of adverse perinatal outcome in congenital cytomegalovirus infection: a retrospective multicenter study. J Perinat Med 2022. https://doi.org/10.1515/jpm-2022-0286.
42. Buca D, Di Mascio D, Rizzo G, et al. Outcome of fetuses with congenital cytomegalovirus infection and normal ultrasound at diagnosis: systematic review and meta-analysis. Ultrasound Obstet Gynecol 2021;57(4):551–9.
43. Picone O, Teissier N, Cordier AG, et al. Detailed in utero ultrasound description of 30 cases of congenital cytomegalovirus infection. Prenat Diagn 2014;34(6): 518–24.
44. Guerra B, Simonazzi G, Puccetti C, et al. Ultrasound prediction of symptomatic congenital cytomegalovirus infection. Am J Obstet Gynecol 2008;198(4): 380.e1–7.
45. Nigro G, La Torre R, Pentimalli H, et al. Regression of fetal cerebral abnormalities by primary cytomegalovirus infection following hyperimmunoglobulin therapy. Prenat Diagn 2008;28(6):512–7.
46. Jacquemard F, Yamamoto M, Costa JM, et al. Maternal administration of valaciclovir in symptomatic intrauterine cytomegalovirus infection. BJOG 2007; 114(9):1113–21.
47. Leruez-Ville M, Ghout I, Bussières L, et al. In utero treatment of congenital cytomegalovirus infection with valacyclovir in a multicenter, open-label, phase II study. Am J Obstet Gynecol 2016;215(4):462.e1–10.

48. Codaccioni C, Vauloup-Fellous C, Letamendia E, et al. Case report on early treatment with valaciclovir after maternal primary cytomegalovirus infection. J Gynecol Obstet Hum Reprod 2019;48(4):287–9.
49. Hold PM, Wong CF, Dhanda RK, et al. Successful renal transplantation during pregnancy. Am J Transplant 2005;5(9):2315–7.
50. Nicloux M, Peterman L, Parodi M, et al. Outcome and management of newborns with congenital cytomegalovirus infection. Arch Pediatr 2020;27(3):160–5.
51. Kurath S, Halwachs-Baumann G, Müller W, et al. Transmission of cytomegalovirus via breast milk to the prematurely born infant: a systematic review. Clin Microbiol Infect 2010;16(8):1172–8.
52. Coclite E, Di Natale C, Nigro G. Congenital and perinatal cytomegalovirus lung infection. J Matern Fetal Neonatal Med 2013;26(17):1671–5.
53. Bimboese P, Kadambari S, Tabrizi SN, et al. Postnatal cytomegalovirus infection of preterm and very-low-birth-weight infants through maternal breast milk: does it matter? Pediatr Infect Dis J 2022;41(4):343–51.
54. Bardanzellu F, Fanos V, Reali A. Human breast milk-acquired cytomegalovirus infection: certainties, doubts and perspectives. Curr Pediatr Rev 2019;15(1):30–41.
55. Davis NL, King CC, Kourtis AP. Cytomegalovirus infection in pregnancy. Birth Defects Res 2017;109(5):336–46.
56. Goderis J, De Leenheer E, Smets K, et al. Hearing loss and congenital CMV infection: a systematic review. Pediatrics 2014;134(5):972–82.

Safety and Effectiveness of Maternal COVID-19 Vaccines Among Pregnant People and Infants

Katherine E. Fleming-Dutra, MD[a],[*],[1],
Lauren Head Zauche, PhD, MSN[b],[1], Lauren E. Roper, MPH[a],
Sascha R. Ellington, PhD[c], Christine K. Olson, MD[b],[d],
Andrea J. Sharma, PhD[b],[d], Kate R. Woodworth, MD[e],
Naomi Tepper, MD[d],[e], Fiona Havers, MD[a],[d], Sara E. Oliver, MD[a],[d],
Evelyn Twentyman, MD[a], Tara C. Jatlaoui, MD[d],[f]

KEYWORDS

- COVID-19 vaccine • Pregnancy • Infants • mRNA vaccines • Vaccine effectiveness
- Vaccine safety • Maternal vaccination

KEY POINTS

- Available evidence demonstrates that COVID-19 vaccination during pregnancy is safe and is not associated with adverse pregnancy or infant outcomes.
- Reactogenicity to COVID-19 vaccines is similar for pregnant people and nonpregnant women of reproductive age for both doses in the primary messenger RNA (mRNA) vaccine series.
- Effectiveness of mRNA COVID-19 vaccines is similar in pregnant people and nonpregnant women of similar age for prevention of SARS-CoV-2 infection and hospitalizations.
- Maternal COVID-19 vaccination during pregnancy reduces the risk of SARS-CoV-2 infection and COVID-19–associated hospitalization in infants younger than 6 months.

Continued

[a] National Center for Immunization and Respiratory Diseases, Centers for Disease Control and Prevention, 1600 Clifton Road NE, Mailstop H24-9 Atlanta, GA 30329, USA; [b] Division of Healthcare Quality Promotion, National Center for Emerging and Zoonotic Infectious Diseases, Centers for Disease Control and Prevention, Atlanta, GA, USA; [c] Division of Reproductive Health, National Center for Chronic Disease Prevention and Health Promotion, Centers for Disease Control and Prevention, Atlanta, GA, USA; [d] U.S. Public Health Service Commissioned Corps, Atlanta, GA, USA; [e] Division of Birth Defects and Infant Disorders, National Center on Birth Defects and Developmental Disabilities, Centers for Disease Control and Prevention, Atlanta, GA, USA; [f] Immunization Services Division, National Center for Immunization and Respiratory Diseases, Centers for Disease Control and Prevention, Atlanta, GA, USA
[1] Drs K.E. Fleming-Dutra and L.H. Zauche contributed equally to this article.
* Corresponding author.
E-mail address: ftu2@cdc.gov

Obstet Gynecol Clin N Am 50 (2023) 279–297
https://doi.org/10.1016/j.ogc.2023.02.003
0889-8545/23/Published by Elsevier Inc.

obgyn.theclinics.com

Continued

- The effectiveness of maternal monovalent mRNA COVID-19 vaccination was lower for infections and hospitalizations in both pregnant people and infants during predominance of the Omicron variant than during predominance of prior SARS-CoV-2 variants.

INTRODUCTION

Maternal vaccination is a safe and effective strategy to prevent morbidity and mortality from vaccine-preventable diseases both among pregnant people and through transplacental transfer of antibodies, among infants after birth.[1] Influenza, pertussis, and COVID-19 vaccines are all recommended for pregnant persons.[2–4] Influenza vaccine is recommended for everyone age 6 months and older, including pregnant people, every influenza season, and maternal influenza vaccination provides protection for the mother during pregnancy and the infant after birth.[2] In comparison, acellular pertussis vaccine (Tdap) is recommended for pregnant people during every pregnancy, optimally between 27 and 36 weeks gestation, with the goal of maximizing protection for the infant in the first few months after birth.[4] COVID-19 can cause severe disease in pregnant people. Compared with nonpregnant women of similar age, pregnant people with COVID-19 are at increased risk for admission to the intensive care unit (ICU) and for requiring mechanical ventilation and extracorporeal membrane oxygen support.[5] COVID-19 during pregnancy also increases the risk of adverse pregnancy outcomes, including preterm birth, stillbirth, infant neonatal ICU admission, and rarely, maternal and neonatal death.[5] Pregnant people have been eligible for COVID-19 vaccination in the United States since the initial Emergency Use Authorizations (EUA) in December 2020 and were initially given the option of vaccination[6]; however, they were not included in initial clinical trials.[7–10] Based on accumulating data on COVID-19 safety and effectiveness, in August 2021, the Centers for Disease Control and Prevention (CDC) strengthened its recommendations for COVID-19 vaccination of all pregnant people.[11]

COVID-19 vaccination during pregnancy, regardless of trimester of exposure, is associated with detectable antibodies in maternal sera, umbilical cord blood, and infant sera at delivery that may provide protection to infants against COVID-19.[12,13] Antibodies after vaccination in maternal and cord blood at delivery demonstrate neutralizing responses, and antibodies in infant sera can persist through early infancy, with one study detecting antibodies to at least 12 weeks of age.[13] Moreover, infants younger than 6 months are the only population in the United States not currently eligible for COVID-19 vaccination. Infants may be hospitalized and may become critically ill.[14,15] Among infants younger than 6 months, COVID-19 causes a similar to higher burden of hospitalizations than influenza,[16] which has long been recognized as a cause of severe respiratory disease in this population.[17]

Because pregnant people were excluded from the COVID-19 vaccine clinical trials, postauthorization studies and surveillance have been important to inform vaccine safety and effectiveness among pregnant people. Several reviews, including 3 recent reports (of which 2 were meta-analyses), have covered COVID-19 vaccine safety and effectiveness in pregnancy,[18–20] and recently new evidence has emerged on the vaccine effectiveness of monovalent COVID-19 booster doses among pregnant people and the effects of maternal COVID-19 vaccination among infants. The objective of this review is to provide an update on COVID-19 vaccination coverage among pregnant people and an overview of the evidence on COVID-19 vaccine safety and effectiveness in pregnant people for vaccines authorized or approved for use in the United States, with further discussion of booster doses and potential benefits in infants.

COVID-19 VACCINE RECOMMENDATIONS AND COVERAGE IN PREGNANT PEOPLE IN THE UNITED STATES

CDC recommends everyone ages 6 months and older, including pregnant people, stay up to date with COVID-19 vaccines recommended for their age group.[3] As of October 12, 2022, people ages 5 years and older are recommended to receive one updated (bivalent) Pfizer-BioNTech or Moderna messenger RNA (mRNA) booster.[3] Bivalent mRNA boosters contain mRNA encoding the spike protein from both the Omicron (BA.4/BA.5) SARS-CoV-2 variants and the ancestral (or original) SARS-CoV-2 strain, whereas the original (monovalent) mRNA vaccines only contain mRNA encoding the ancestral strain spike protein. The bivalent booster dose should be administered at least 2 months after completion of the primary series or the last monovalent booster dose. For those ages 18 years and older who have completed a primary series but not a booster, Novavax monovalent COVID-19 vaccine is available as an alternative for those who cannot or will not pursue bivalent booster vaccination.[21] CDC's guidance on staying up to date with COVID-19 vaccines and coadministration with non-COVID-19 vaccines applies to everyone, including pregnant people.[3] COVID-19 vaccines may be administered without regard to timing of other vaccines, and this includes simultaneous administration of COVID-19 vaccine and other vaccines, such as influenza and Tdap vaccines, on the same day. However, there are additional considerations if administering an orthopoxvirus vaccine (which is used for the prevention of monkeypox and smallpox); this guidance is available on CDC's Web site.[3]

Data collected from CDC's National Immunization Survey-Adult COVID-19 Module during August 28 to September 30, 2022 indicated that 25.6% (95% confidence interval [CI] 16.6%–34.5%) of pregnant people had not yet received any COVID-19 vaccine, 72.0% (95% CI 62.9%–81.1%) had completed a primary series, and 4.3% (95% CI 0.0%–8.7%) were up to date with a primary series or bivalent booster, when indicated.[22] In comparison, 16.0% (95% CI 14.6%–17.3%) of women ages 18 to 49 years who were not pregnant, trying to become pregnant, or breastfeeding remained unvaccinated, 81.6% (95% CI 80.2%–83.1%) had completed a primary series, and 3.6% (95% CI 2.9%–4.3%) were up to date with a primary series or bivalent booster, when indicated.[22] These data indicate that opportunities remain to increase primary series COVID-19 vaccination and bivalent booster uptake among pregnant people.

SAFETY OF COVID-19 VACCINES IN PREGNANT PEOPLE AND THEIR INFANTS

Vaccine safety is essential to ensure the well-being of vaccine recipients and trust in regulatory and public health agencies. All vaccines undergo rigorous testing through several phases of clinical trials before authorization or approval for use in the general population. However, because pregnant people were excluded from initial trials, initial safety data came from developmental and reproductive toxicity animal studies and from a very small sample of participants who became pregnant during the preauthorization vaccine trials.[23] Animal studies did not identify any safety concerns for female fertility or embryonal or fetal development.[24,25] No safety concerns were identified in the 23 participants who became pregnant in the monovalent Pfizer-BioNTech mRNA COVID-19 vaccine (BNT162b2) trial or the 12 participants who became pregnant in the monovalent Moderna mRNA COVID-19 vaccine (mRNA-1273) trial.[24,25] Because mRNA vaccines have been the most widely used, most safety data to date in pregnant people come from postauthorization safety monitoring and observational studies examining monovalent mRNA vaccines, specifically primary series vaccination. Included studies are detailed in Supplementary Table 1.

Local and Systemic Reactions

Monitoring the reactogenicity to vaccination is important for establishing and understanding a vaccine's safety profile. Because vaccines stimulate an immune response, it is common for individuals to experience local adverse events following vaccination such as pain, redness, rash, or swelling around the injection site, as well as systemic adverse events, such as fever, myalgia, arthralgia, headache, and nausea or vomiting.

The v-safe after vaccination health checker is a smartphone–based active surveillance system developed by CDC to monitor for adverse events and reactogenicity following COVID-19 vaccination.[26] Vaccinated individuals voluntarily enroll in v-safe and receive text messages with weblinks to online surveys that assess for adverse events, severity of symptoms, and health impact of symptoms. To identify people who received a COVID-19 vaccine while pregnant, v-safe surveys include a question inquiring about pregnancy status for nonmale participants. Preliminary findings from 16,982 v-safe participants who identified as pregnant and completed a survey about reactions on postvaccination day 1 during December 14, 2020 and February 28, 2021 demonstrated that local and systemic reactions following vaccination with BNT162b2 and mRNA-1273 vaccines were common after each dose but were more frequently reported after dose 2 compared with dose 1.[26] The symptoms most commonly reported the day after vaccination included injection-site pain (88.1% postdose 1, 91.9% postdose 2), fatigue (29.6% postdose 1, 71.5% postdose 2), headache (18.1% postdose 1, 55.4% postdose 2), myalgia (11.6% postdose 1, 54.1% postdose 2), chills (4.1% postdose 1, 36.7% postdose 2), and fever (4.2% postdose 1, 34.6% postdose 2). The prevalence of these symptoms and higher reactogenicity after dose 2 were similar to those of nonpregnant women of reproductive age. Systemic reactions were reported more frequently among nonpregnant women of reproductive age except for nausea and vomiting, which was reported more frequently in pregnant people.[26]

Results from other surveillance systems have observed similar reactogenicity profiles for the monovalent mRNA COVID-19 vaccines. In a prospective cohort study of 1012 pregnant people from the Swiss COVI-PREG registry, 35.3% and 67.3% reported a systemic reaction after dose 1 and dose 2, respectively; systemic reactions were primarily fatigue, headache, and myalgia and were more common with mRNA-1273 compared with BNT162b2.[27] Results from a case-control study of 390 pregnant people and 260 nonpregnant women who all received BNT162b2 in Israel demonstrated that myalgia, arthralgia, and headache occurred more frequently among the nonpregnant control group, but paresthesia (tingling sensation) was more common among pregnant people compared with nonpregnant people postdose 2 (4.6% vs 1.2%, $P < .001$).[28] Incidence of uterine contractions (1.3% for dose 1, 6.4% for dose 2) and vaginal bleeding (0.3% postdose 1, 1.5% postdose 2) were low but were more common after dose 2; uterine contractions did not result in preterm birth for any pregnant people in the study.[28] However, this study did not include unvaccinated pregnant people and could not compare with the baseline risk of these events.[28]

Severe adverse events following vaccination in pregnant people are much less common compared with local and systemic reactions. In a report from the Canadian National Vaccine Safety Network, 226 (4.0%) of 5597 vaccinated pregnant people reported a significant health event, which was defined as a new or worsening health event sufficient to cause work or school absenteeism, medical consultation, or to prevent normal daily activities after dose 1 of an mRNA COVID-19 vaccine.[29] After dose 2, 7.3% reported a significant health event. The most common significant health events were malaise, myalgia, and headache.[29] Fewer than 1% of participants experienced a serious health event, defined as an event resulting in an emergency department or hospital visit.[29] These findings were consistent with electronic health data from the Vaccine Safety Datalink, a collaborative project between CDC and 9 integrated health care organizations in the United States to monitor vaccine safety.[30] Of 45,232 pregnant people who had received a COVID-19 vaccine immediately before or during pregnancy, fewer than 1% experienced symptoms for which they needed to seek medical care. Serious acute adverse events, including cerebral venous sinus thrombosis, encephalitis or myelitis, Guillain-Barré syndrome, myocarditis, pericarditis, or pulmonary embolism, did not occur more frequently in vaccinated pregnant people compared with nonvaccinated pregnant people.

During December 14, 2020 and October 31, 2021, a total of 3462 reports of adverse events in pregnant people who received a COVID-19 primary series dose (91.8% received an mRNA vaccine, 7.9% received Ad26.COV2.S [Janssen] vaccine) were submitted to the Vaccine Adverse Event Reporting System (VAERS), a passive surveillance system in the United States.[31] A total of 621 reports (17.9%) were categorized as serious, including 8 maternal deaths and 12 neonatal deaths. Medical record review for cases in which records could be obtained did not identify any concerning patterns for cause or probable cause of death that could be attributed to vaccination.[31] VAERS also received 323 reports of adverse events in pregnant people who received a monovalent mRNA vaccine booster dose from September 22, 2021 through March 24, 2022; 72 (22.3%) were coded as serious, most of which were spontaneous abortions (n = 56).[32] Review of VAERS reports did not identify any unexpected reporting of any adverse events compared with other vaccines in VAERS for either the COVID-19 vaccine primary series or the booster dose.[31,32]

Spontaneous Abortion

Spontaneous abortion (SAB), that is, pregnancy loss before 20 weeks gestation, is a common pregnancy outcome, affecting 11% to 22% of all recognized pregnancies.[33,34] Concern about the risk of SAB may be a barrier to early maternal vaccination. Because the underlying risk of SAB varies by week of pregnancy, it is essential that time-varying exposure methods be considered to minimize bias in studies assessing SAB after vaccination.[35] To date, no surveillance systems or studies have identified any association between SAB and COVID-19 vaccination.[19,29,36–39]

Participants in CDC's v-safe after vaccination health checker[SM] who reported they were pregnant at the time of vaccination or shortly thereafter were invited to participate in CDC's COVID-19 Vaccine Pregnancy Registry. The pregnancy registry reported a 14.1% (95% CI 12.1%–16.1%) cumulative risk of SAB from 6 to less than 20 weeks gestation among a cohort of 2456 pregnant people who received at least one dose of an mRNA COVID-19 vaccine 30 days before their last menstrual period through 19 weeks 6 days gestation.[36] After age-standardization with a reference population, the cumulative risk of SAB was 12.8% (95% CI 10.8%–14.8%), consistent with published estimates of underlying risk of SAB in reference populations.[33,34,36] However, this analysis was limited by several factors, including no control group and a sample that consisted of mostly non-Hispanic White health care personnel.

A meta-analysis by Prasad and colleagues[19] that pooled results from 2 comparative studies with time-varying exposures[38,39] found no association between COVID-19 vaccine and SAB (odds ratio [OR]: 1.00, 95% CI 0.92 to 1.09). In another retrospective cohort study, the rate of first trimester SAB among 927 vaccinated pregnant people in Romania was 13.4%.[37] There were no increased odds of first trimester SAB for those who received BNT162b2 (adjusted odds ratio [aOR]: 1.04, 95% CI 0.91 to 1.12) or mRNA-1273 (aOR: 1.02, 95% CI 0.89–1.08) compared with those not vaccinated.[37] These results taken together suggest that COVID-19 vaccination does not increase the risk of SAB.

Stillbirth

Stillbirth, or intrauterine fetal demise occurring at or after 20 weeks gestation, is a devastating pregnancy outcome that occurs in approximately 5.7 per 1000 births in the United States.[40] Recent reports have demonstrated that SARS-CoV-2 infection during pregnancy is associated with an almost 2-fold increased risk of stillbirth.[5,41] In contrast, studies assessing COVID-19 vaccination during pregnancy have not identified an increased risk of stillbirth following vaccination.

In a systematic review and meta-analysis that included 7 studies of 66,067 vaccinated and 425,624 unvaccinated pregnant people, receipt of an mRNA COVID-19 vaccination during pregnancy was associated with a 15% reduction in the odds of stillbirth (OR: 0.85, 95% CI 0.73–0.99).[19] These results were similar to those of another meta-analysis that included 5 studies (3 of which were included in Prasad and colleagues) of 31,796 vaccinated and 135,652 unvaccinated pregnant people and identified a 27% reduction in the odds of stillbirth among those vaccinated with any COVID-19 vaccine (OR: 0.73, 95% CI 0.57–0.94), although it is important to note that the definition of stillbirth varied among the studies included in the meta-analysis.[20] In a large population-based registry in Norway and Sweden with 28,506 vaccinated singleton pregnancies and 129,015 nonvaccinated singleton pregnancies, the rate of stillbirths after vaccination was 2.1 per 100,000 pregnancy days, whereas the rate of stillbirths was 2.4 per 100,000 pregnancy days among those unvaccinated (adjusted hazard ratio [aHR]: 0.86, 95% CI 0.63 to 1.17).[42] Similarly, Hui and colleagues found lower odds of stillbirths among 17,365 mRNA-vaccinated singleton pregnancies compared with 15,171 unvaccinated singleton pregnancies in an Australian-based registry (aOR: 0.18, 95% CI 0.09–0.37).[43] The protective effect of vaccination is likely partially due to the prevention of severe COVID-19 illness, which is associated with stillbirth, but it is also possible that this result may in part be due to confounding. Vaccinated people in this study may have been healthier overall and seemed to have better access and adherence to prenatal care (with higher rates of receiving gestational diabetes screening) than unvaccinated people.[43]

Gestational Conditions

Development of conditions during pregnancy such as hypertensive disorders or gestational diabetes has significant implications for the health of both the mother and the fetus. Evidence from 4 retrospective cohort studies, 1 case-control study, and a meta-analysis suggests no increased risk of hypertensive disorders of pregnancy or gestational diabetes among those who received a COVID-19 vaccine during pregnancy compared with those who were unvaccinated.[19,28,44–47] Dick and colleagues reported on an Israeli cohort of 5618 pregnant participants, of which 2305 participants had received an mRNA COVID-19 vaccine in the second or third trimester.[44] Compared with unvaccinated participants, those vaccinated had no increased odds of a hypertensive disorder of pregnancy (aOR: 0.71, 95% CI 0.33–1.54 for second trimester vaccination; aOR: 0.83, 95% CI 0.45–1.55 for third trimester vaccination) or gestational diabetes (aOR: 1.21, 95% CI 0.93–1.58 for second trimester vaccination; aOR: 0.99, 95% CI: 0.77–1.27 for third trimester vaccination).[44] Similarly, there were no increased odds of preeclampsia or eclampsia (aOR: 1.17, 95% CI 0.84–1.61) among a cohort of 913 pregnant people who received a BNT162b2 vaccine during pregnancy compared with 3486 unvaccinated pregnant people.[47]

In addition, no studies identified any increased risk of oligohydramnios,[28,47] polyhydramnios,[28,47] nonvertex presentation,[47] thromboembolism,[46] stroke,[46] or antepartum bleeding[48] among vaccinated compared with unvaccinated pregnant people.

Delivery Complications

COVID-19 vaccination during pregnancy has not been associated with increased risk of any adverse peripartum outcomes compared with unvaccinated pregnant people, including cesarean delivery (overall and emergency),[49] postpartum hemorrhage,[28,44,46,47,49–51] chorioamnionitis,[50,51] endometritis,[28,51] placental abruption,[28,47] nonreassuring fetal heart tones,[47] vacuum or forceps delivery,[28,47] low 5-min APGAR score (<7),[49] maternal ICU admission,[46,49,51] or meconium-stained amniotic fluid.[45,47] In a meta-analysis of 5 studies, receipt of any COVID-19 vaccine during pregnancy was not associated with either cesarean delivery (OR: 1.05, 95% CI 0.93–0.1.20) or postpartum hemorrhage (OR: 0.95, 95% CI 0.83–1.07).[20] Meta-analysis of 3 studies also showed no increased risk for chorioamnionitis among vaccinated pregnant people (OR: 1.06, 95% CI 0.86–1.31).[20] Two studies found a decreased odds of meconium-stained fluid among vaccinated people compared with unvaccinated people (aOR: 0.63, 95% CI: 0.49–0.83; aOR: 0.64, 95% CI: 0.43–0.96),[45,47] and one study identified decreased odds of nonreassuring fetal heart tones during delivery (aOR: 0.64, 95% CI 0.44, 0.90).[47]

Most of the studies that investigated peripartum outcomes included pregnant people vaccinated during any trimester during pregnancy. Dick and colleagues compared peripartum outcomes of people vaccinated in the second and third trimesters with unvaccinated pregnant people and found no significant differences in the odds of low APGAR score (<7) at 5 minutes, cesarean delivery, or postpartum hemorrhage by trimester of vaccination.[44] Similarly, Rottenstreich and colleagues investigated adverse peripartum outcomes in pregnant people vaccinated in the third trimester by creating a composite adverse maternal outcome variable, defined as experiencing at least one of the following: chorioamnionitis, postpartum hemorrhage, endometritis, blood transfusion, cesarean delivery, ICU admission, or extended length of stay (>5 days for vaginal delivery or >7 days for cesarean).[51] The investigators reported that receipt of COVID-19 vaccination at greater than 24 weeks gestation was not associated with the maternal composite adverse outcome (aOR: 0.8, 95% CI 0.61–1.03) compared with no receipt of the COVID-19 vaccine.[51]

Placental Histopathology

The effect of SARS-CoV-2 infection on placental histopathology is a topic of investigation[52]; it remains unknown whether the COVID-19 vaccine affects the placenta. Two studies were identified that compared placental histopathology of pregnant people who had been vaccinated with a COVID-19 vaccine and unvaccinated pregnant people in the United States.[53,54] In a cross-sectional study of 200 pregnant people, of which 84 people received a COVID-19 vaccine during pregnancy, there was no increased odds of decidual arteriopathy (aOR: 0.75, 95% CI 0.3–1.9), fetal vascular malperfusion (aOR: 0.85, 95% CI 0.27–2.7), or low-grade chronic villitis (aOR: 1.6, 95% CI 0.62–4.2).[53] There was decreased odds of high-grade chronic villitis (aOR: 0.31, 95% CI 0.1–0.97).[53] Similarly, Boelig and colleagues reported no significant differences in the odds of placental maternal vascular malperfusion (aOR: 0.61, 95% CI

0.22–1.68) comparing 49 vaccinated pregnant people with 198 unvaccinated pregnant people in a retrospective cohort study.[54] However, in this same study, those who were unvaccinated but had COVID-19 in pregnancy (n = 59) had significantly higher odds of placental maternal vascular malperfusion than those without COVID-19 (aOR: 2.34, 95% CI 1.16–4.73).[54] These results suggest that SARS-CoV-2 infection, but not COVID-19 vaccination, affects placental vascular pathology.

Preterm birth, small for gestational age, neonatal intensive care unit admission

Previous studies have suggested that SARS-CoV-2 infection during pregnancy significantly increases the risk of preterm birth (delivery <37 weeks gestation), small for gestational age (SGA) (<10% in birth weight for sex), and infant admission to the neonatal intensive care unit (NICU).[5,55] Although multiple studies have examined the risk of preterm birth, SGA, and NICU admission following receipt of COVID-19 vaccination in pregnancy, none have detected any increased risks.[19,20] Methodologically, investigation of preterm birth is challenging, as analytical techniques to adjust for time-varying exposure must be considered to minimize biased results.[35]

In a retrospective cohort study from the Vaccine Safety Datalink, risks for preterm birth and SGA at birth among 10,064 vaccinated and 36,015 unvaccinated pregnant people were compared, accounting for time-dependent vaccine exposures and propensity to be vaccinated based on maternal age, race and ethnicity, adequacy of prenatal care, comorbidities, neighborhood poverty rate, state-level percentage of positive COVID-19 test results, and site.[56] COVID-19 vaccination during pregnancy was not associated with either preterm birth (aHR: 0.91, 95% CI 0.82–1.01) or SGA (aHR: 0.95 95% CI 0.87–1.03). After stratifying by second and third trimester vaccination, results consistently showed no increased risk.[56] A large population-based retrospective study in Norway and Sweden that accounted for time-varying exposure also found no increased risk of preterm birth (aHR: 0.98, 95% CI 0.91–1.05) or increased odds of SGA (aOR: 0.97, 95% CI 0.90–1.04) or NICU admission (aOR: 0.97, 95% CI 0.86, 1.10).[42] Results for SGA and NICU admission were similar in a sensitivity analysis restricting the sample to only term births.[42] Furthermore, in a meta-analysis with 6 studies, receipt of a COVID-19 vaccine in pregnancy was associated with a 12% reduction in the odds of infant NICU admission (OR: 0.88, 95% CI 0.80–0.97).[20] This meta-analysis also pooled results of 7 studies that examined preterm birth and 6 studies that examined SGA; COVID-19 vaccination was not significantly associated with either preterm birth (OR: 0.89, 95% CI 0.76–1.04) or SGA (OR: 0.99, 95% CI 0.94–1.04).[20]

Some studies restricted analyses to investigate risk of preterm birth or SGA based on trimester of first vaccine receipt. First trimester vaccination exposure did not increase risk of preterm birth (RR: 0.87, 95% CI 0.67–1.12) or SGA (RR: 1.14, 95% CI 0.92–1.40) in a retrospective cohort study from Israel; no significant differences for early preterm or moderately preterm births were detected.[57] Similarly, Theiler and colleagues found no significant increase in the prevalence of preterm birth at less than 24 weeks, 24 to less than 32 weeks, and 32 to less than 37 weeks gestation.[46] Second or third trimester vaccination exposure was also not associated with increased odds of SGA at birth (aOR: 0.73, 95% CI 0.52–1.03 for second trimester; aOR: 0.85, 95% CI 0.64–1.13 for third trimester) in another retrospective cohort study from Israel.[44] However, second trimester vaccination was associated with increased odds of preterm birth (aOR: 1.49, 95% CI 1.11–2.01); though no preterm births occurred within 2 weeks after vaccination and most of these births were after 35 weeks gestation. In this same study, third trimester vaccination was associated with decreased odds of preterm birth (aOR: 0.49, 95% CI 0.34–0.71); the study investigators note that their results may differ from other studies due to their inability to control for several risk factors for preterm birth.[44]

Infant Hospitalization and Infant Mortality

All-cause infant hospitalization and infant mortality are important outcomes to monitor in infants of people vaccinated during pregnancy. To date, there are limited studies available that have investigated these outcomes. In a population-based retrospective cohort study of 24,288 infants in Israel, risk of neonatal hospitalization was not significantly different among infants prenatally exposed to BNT162b2 in the first trimester (risk ratio [RR]: 0.86, 95% CI 0.67–1.09) or during any trimester in pregnancy (RR: 0.99, 95% CI 0.88–1.12) compared with unexposed infants.[57] In addition, compared with unexposed infants, there was no increased risk for postneonatal hospitalization for either prenatal exposure in the first trimester (RR: 0.95, 95% CI 0.84–1.07) or any trimester in pregnancy (RR: 0.78, 95% CI 0.54–1.09).[57] Infant mortality rates were low for both infants exposed prenatally to BNT162b2 and for infants unexposed prenatally (0.1% in both groups); no difference was observed in mortality for infants exposed in the first trimester to the vaccine compared with those who were not exposed to the vaccine (RR: 0.69, 95% CI 0.14–2.41).[57]

Perinatal mortality, which is inclusive of both stillbirths and neonatal deaths, was compared between pregnant people in Scotland who received any COVID-19 vaccine during pregnancy (regardless of infection status) and those who had SARS-CoV-2 infection during pregnancy (regardless of vaccination status).[58] Among those who received a COVID-19 vaccine during pregnancy, the perinatal mortality rate was 4.3 (95% CI 2.9–6.4) per 1000 births compared with 8.0 (95% CI 5.0–12.8) and 22.6 (95% CI 12.9–38.5) among those who had SARS-CoV-2 infection (regardless of vaccination status) during pregnancy or within 28 days of delivery, respectively; all perinatal deaths occurring after SARS-CoV-2 infection occurred in pregnant people who were unvaccinated.[58]

Congenital Anomalies

Few studies have investigated the risk of congenital anomalies among vaccinated pregnant people. Ruderman and colleagues retrospectively compared the odds of a fetal structural anomaly identified through ultrasonography for 1149 pregnant people vaccinated with either an mRNA vaccine or Ad26.COV2.S (Janssen) vaccine 30 days before conception through 14 weeks gestation with 2007 pregnant people who were either unvaccinated or received a COVID-19 vaccine after 14 weeks gestation; the first trimester (<14 weeks gestation) is a period of organogenesis when impacts of exposures on the development of structural birth defects would be more likely to occur.[59] COVID-19 vaccination (≥1 dose of any COVID-19 vaccine) was not associated with the presence of a fetal structural defect identified on ultrasonography (aOR: 1.05; 95% CI 0.72–1.54).[59] Findings were similar even after narrowing the window of exposure to 2 to 10 weeks gestation (aOR: 0.96, 95% CI 0.63–1.45).[59] A limitation of this analysis is that birth defect surveillance typically relies on postnatal confirmation and collection of data through the first year of life rather than ultrasonography.[60] However, similar results were reported in 2 large population-based retrospective cohort studies that evaluated congenital anomalies postnatally among infants born to pregnant people who were vaccinated.[43,57] Data from a large population-based study conducted in Israel found no increased risk of overall congenital anomalies (adjusted risk ratio [aRR]: 0.69, 95% CI 0.44 to 1.04) and a decreased risk of a major congenital heart anomaly (aRR: 0.46, 95% CI 0.24–0.82) diagnosed in the first month of life among infants who were exposed to BNT162b2 in the first trimester (n = 2021) compared with those unexposed (n = 3580).[57] In an Australian registry of 17,365 singleton infants exposed to mRNA vaccines prenatally, the odds of a congenital anomaly diagnosed at birth were lower compared with those not exposed to a vaccine prenatally (aOR: 0.72, 95% CI 0.56–0.94). However, after restricting the sample to those vaccinated less than 20 weeks gestation, the odds of a congenital anomaly were the same among pregnant people who did and did not receive a COVID-19 vaccine (aOR: 0.80, 95% CI 0.57–1.13).[43] Although reassuring that no increase in congenital anomalies has been detected in infants through 1 month of age, birth defect surveillance typically goes through 1 year of life, so additional follow-up will be needed to confirm these findings.

Safety Summary

COVID-19 vaccination during pregnancy does not seem to increase the risk for any adverse pregnancy, maternal, or neonatal outcomes. The reactogenicity profile of mRNA vaccines is similar among pregnant people and nonpregnant women of reproductive age, although there was a lower incidence of systemic effects following vaccination among pregnant people. Data from national registries and observational cohort studies suggest no increased risk of spontaneous abortion and a decreased risk of stillbirth following COVID-19 vaccination in pregnancy. Furthermore, evidence suggests no increased risk of congenital anomalies among those vaccinated in the first trimester compared with unvaccinated pregnant people. Risks of preterm birth, SGA, NICU admission, infant hospitalization, placental pathologic findings, and pregnancy and obstetric complications, including gestational diabetes, hypertensive disorders, and nonelective cesarean delivery, were similar between vaccinated and unvaccinated pregnant people. Risk of perinatal mortality was higher among people who had COVID-19 during pregnancy compared with those who were vaccinated and did not have COVID-19 during pregnancy. Overall, these results on maternal and neonatal outcomes were observed consistently across studies regardless of type of vaccine and timing of vaccine exposure. These postauthorization safety data on a variety of pregnancy, maternal, and neonatal outcomes support recommendations for COVID-19 vaccination during pregnancy and provide reassurance to pregnant people and their health care providers that COVID-19 vaccines are safe.

EFFECTIVENESS OF MATERNAL COVID-19 VACCINATION

Data regarding effectiveness of COVID-19 vaccines for the prevention of infection and disease among pregnant people and their infants are only available from observational studies conducted after vaccine introduction, and data remain limited. For vaccines currently authorized or approved in the United States, vaccine effectiveness (VE) data among pregnant people and infants are currently only available for the monovalent mRNA COVID-19 vaccines. Here, the authors review the evidence from studies assessing effectiveness of monovalent mRNA vaccines in pregnant people or infants younger than 6 months against laboratory-confirmed SARS-CoV-2 infection, symptomatic or medically attended COVID-19, COVID-19-associated hospitalization, and severe or critical COVID-19. Studies estimating the effect of COVID-19 vaccines on adverse pregnancy outcomes have done so primarily to assess vaccine safety and thus are covered in the safety section of this review. Studies assessing VE against death among pregnant people and young infants are not available due to the rarity of this outcome.

For Outcomes Occurring Among Pregnant People

Vaccine effectiveness for SARS-COV-2 infection

Two studies from Israel and one from Qatar conducted soon after COVID-19 vaccine rollout examined effectiveness of 2 doses of mRNA vaccines in pregnant people and showed high VE against SARS-CoV-2 infection (Supplementary Table 2),[61–63] and these results were similar to those in the general populations of those countries.[64,65] Goldshtein and colleagues conducted an observational cohort study among pregnant people in Israel during the first 4 months of vaccine rollout (December 19, 2020 to April 11, 2021) and found effectiveness of 2 BNT162b2 doses for laboratory-confirmed infection was high at 28 days or more after dose 1 (ie, >7 days after dose 2): VE 78% (95% CI 57%–89%).[61] Another Israeli cohort study by Dagan and colleagues conducted among pregnant people during December 2020 to June 2021 also demonstrated high VE for 2 doses of BNT162b2 during days 7 to 56 after the second dose for laboratory-confirmed infection (VE 96% [95% CI 89%–100%]), symptomatic COVID-19 (VE 97% [95% CI 91%–100%]), and hospitalization (VE 89% [95% CI 43%–100%]).[62] These results were also similar to previously published estimates from the same investigators among the general Israeli population ages 16 years or older during a similar time frame (December 20, 2020 to February 1, 2021), in which VE for laboratory-confirmed infection was 92% (95% CI 88%–95%), symptomatic COVID-19 94% (95% CI 87%–98%), and hospitalization 87% (95% CI 55%–100%).[64]

A study by Butt and colleagues from Qatar, using data from December 30, 2020 to May 30, 2021 and conducted during circulation of the SARS-CoV-2 Alpha and Beta variants, also found that VE of 2 doses of mRNA vaccines (including both BNT162b2 and mRNA-1273) for infection in pregnant people was high at 14 or more days after the second dose.[63] Using data from the same study population of pregnant people, Butt and colleagues estimated that VE for infection was 87.6% (95% CI 44.1%–97.2%) using a cohort analysis and 86.8% (95% CI 47.5%–98.5%) using a test-negative, case-control analysis.[63] These results were also similar to results among the general population of Qatar in which VE for laboratory-confirmed infection with the Alpha variant was 89.5% (95% CI 85.9%–92.3%) and for Beta variant infection was 75.0% (95% CI 70.5%–78.9%) at 14 or more days after the second dose.[65]

Vaccine effectiveness for COVID-19–associated emergency department and urgent care visits and hospitalizations

Two studies, one from the United States and another from Israel, have assessed VE for medically attended COVID-19, including COVID-19–associated emergency department and urgent care visits and hospitalizations occurring among pregnant people.[66,67] Schrag and colleagues used a test-negative design in CDC's VISION Network to assess effectiveness of monovalent mRNA vaccines for prevention of emergency department and urgent care visits and COVID-19–associated hospitalization occurring during pregnancy.[66] VE was estimated among pregnant people who received at least one dose during pregnancy, pregnant people regardless of whether any doses were received during pregnancy (ie, doses could be received either before or during pregnancy), and for the same outcomes among nonpregnant women ages 18 to 45 years, allowing for comparison of VE estimates among these groups. VE was also stratified by total number of doses received, days since last dose, and by Delta and Omicron variant predominant periods (see Supplementary Table 2). Although power was more limited to assess VE among pregnant people than nonpregnant women, VE estimates were similar among pregnant people and nonpregnant women ages 18 to 45 years, and VE was similar among pregnant people when stratified by doses given during pregnancy versus doses given before or during pregnancy. Furthermore, VE was higher against hospitalization, a more severe outcome, than against emergency department and urgent care visits, a milder outcome. VE was lower during Omicron predominance compared with Delta predominance, and VE waned over time after 2 and 3 doses, particularly during Omicron predominance.[66]

The findings from Schrag and colleagues are similar to those from a publication by Guedalia and colleagues that assessed VE of BNT162b2 for prevention of hospitalization using a population-based cohort study including all pregnant people in Israel who delivered between August 1, 2021 and March 22, 2022.[67] VE was assessed for (1) any hospitalization with a positive SARS-CoV-2 test among pregnant people, which the investigators noted likely reflected VE for infection, as testing was near universal among hospitalized pregnant people; (2) hospitalization with significant disease, defined as having COVID-19 pneumonia; and (3) hospitalization with severe or critical disease, defined as resting respiratory rate greater than 30 breaths per minute, oxygen saturation on room air less than 94%, Pao_2 to Fio_2 ratio of less than 300, mechanical ventilation, clinically severe organ failure, or death. VE was assessed among pregnant people who had received a booster (third) dose and among pregnant people who were eligible for but had yet not received a booster dose (ie, $\geq$150 days after the second dose). They found that among pregnant people in Israel, during Delta variant predominance, VE for any hospitalization (likely reflecting VE for infection) was moderate at 61% (95% CI 51%–69%) at 150 days or more after the second dose, but VE for hospitalization with significant disease and severe disease was high at 150 days or more after the second dose (significant disease VE: 97% [95% CI 92%–99%], severe disease VE: 96% [95% CI 86–99]) and after a booster dose (significant disease VE: 99% [95% CI 93%–100%], severe disease VE: 99% [95% CI 89%–100%], see Supplementary Table 2). However, during Omicron, VE was not significantly different from zero for any of the outcomes at 150 days or more after the second dose. During Omicron, a booster dose increased VE against any hospitalization (likely reflecting VE for infection) to 43% (95% CI 31%–53%) and against significant and severe disease to 97% (95% CI 72%–100%) and 94% (95% CI 43%–99%), respectively. An important caveat to interpreting these results is that VE of 2 doses was measured at 150 days or more after the second dose and thus is reflective of waning, whereas the timing of assessment of VE after the booster dose was not specified but likely reflects a period soon after the booster dose.[67]

Impact of Pregnancy on Vaccine Effectiveness

To address the question of whether pregnancy affected response to vaccine, one study in Norway by Magnus and colleagues examined the relative effectiveness of monovalent mRNA vaccines for prevention of infection, comparing vaccinated pregnant people with vaccinated nonpregnant women who had been pregnant in the year prior but did not receive their COVID-19 vaccines while pregnant or during the postpartum period.[68] They found no differences in the relative effectiveness of the primary series or booster doses between pregnant and nonpregnant people (Supplementary Table 3). During the Omicron predominant period, aHR were 1.03 (95% CI 0.94–1.12) for the comparison of relative effectiveness in pregnant people who received 2 primary series doses during pregnancy compared with nonpregnant women and 1.24 (95% CI 0.84–1.84) for booster dose receipt during pregnancy compared with nonpregnant people.[68]

For Outcomes Occurring Among Infants After Birth

Three studies with four publications have assessed effectiveness of a maternal COVID-19 vaccination for outcomes occurring among infants after birth.[69–72] Two published analyses from CDC's Overcoming COVID-19 network, both by Halasa and colleagues, assessed effectiveness of a maternal monovalent mRNA primary series given during pregnancy for prevention of COVID-19–associated hospitalization among infants younger than 6 months. The first analysis used data from infants hospitalized during July 2021 to January 2022.[69] In the updated analysis, infants younger than 6 months were enrolled from 30 pediatric medical centers in 22 US states from July 2021 to March 2022, a period spanning both Delta and Omicron predominance.[70] As the updated analysis included all data presented in the first analysis, the authors only included results from the updated analysis using data through March 2022. Results from the updated analysis showed that maternal receipt of COVID-19 primary series during pregnancy protected infants younger than 6 months from hospitalization for COVID-19 with an overall VE of 52% (95% CI 33%–65%) for hospitalization and 70% (95% CI 42%–85%) for admission to the ICU (Supplementary Table 4). Among infants, VE for hospitalization was also lower during Omicron predominance (VE 38% [95% CI 8%–58%]) than during Delta (VE 80% [95% CI 60%–90%]). When VE was stratified by timing of vaccination during pregnancy, VE estimates for hospitalization during Delta were not significantly different: 68% (95% CI 19%–87%) for vaccination during the first 20 weeks of pregnancy versus 88% (95% CI 68%–96%) for vaccination after 20 weeks. However, during Omicron predominance, vaccination in the first 20 weeks did not show effectiveness in prevention of hospitalization among infants: (VE 25% [95% CI -26%–56%]), whereas vaccination after 20 weeks was protective (VE 57% [95% CI 25%–75%]).[70]

Two studies assessed maternal vaccination for prevention of SARS-CoV-2 infection in infants after birth (see Supplementary Table 4).[71,72] Carlsen and colleagues used a cohort study including all liveborn infants in Norway from September 1, 2021 to February 28, 2022 to assess effectiveness of maternal COVID-19 vaccination (BNT162b2, mRNA-1273, and ChAdOx1 nCoV-19 [AstraZeneca]) given during the second or third trimesters of pregnancy in prevention of SARS-CoV-2 infection in infants from birth through 3 months of age.[71] This study showed that maternal vaccination with 2 doses (with at least the second dose given during the second or third trimester) provided protection against SARS-CoV-2 infection in infants age up through 3 months, and VE was higher during Delta predominance (VE 71%, [95% CI 56%–81%]) than during Omicron predominance (VE 30% [95% CI 17%–41%]). During Omicron predominance, receipt of a third (booster) dose during the second or third trimester increased VE to 78% (95% CI 57%–88%), but VE estimates were not stratified by time since last dose. Thus, the VE for a third dose may have reflected a shorter time frame after the dose than the VE of a second dose.[71] A publication by Zerbo and colleagues used a cohort design to assess effectiveness of 2 or more doses of monovalent mRNA vaccines for prevention of SARS-CoV-2 infection among infants in northern California younger than 2 months, younger than 4 months, and younger than 6 months during Delta and Omicron periods.[72] During Delta predominance (July 1, 2021 to December 20, 2021), VE for infection among infants was 84% (95% CI 66%–93%) at age less than 2 months, 62% (95% CI 39%–77%) at age less than 4 months, and 56% (95% CI 34%–71%) at age less than 6 months. When stratified by trimester of receipt of the second dose, VE was significant when the second dose was given in the second or third trimester but not during the first trimester. However, during Omicron predominance (December 21, 2021 to May 31, 2022), maternal vaccination was not protective against infection (ie, all VE estimates were not significantly different from zero), including among infants younger than 2 months, younger than 4 months, or younger than 6 months of birth or when stratified by trimester of second dose receipt.[72]

Vaccine Effectiveness Summary

Taken together, results of these studies indicate that effectiveness of mRNA COVID-19 vaccines for prevention of infection and hospitalizations are similar in pregnant people and nonpregnant women of similar age. For these outcomes, time since the last vaccine dose likely affects VE more than whether the vaccine was received during pregnancy. In addition, maternal COVID-19 vaccination during pregnancy protected infants younger than 6 months from infection and hospitalization for COVID-19. The effectiveness of maternal monovalent mRNA COVID-19 vaccines is lower for infections and hospitalizations in both pregnant people and infants during predominance of the Omicron variant than during predominance of prior SARS-CoV-2 variants. The lower VE seen during Omicron predominant time periods is likely due to a combination of factors, including changes in the Omicron spike protein that allowed for immune escape from antibody made against the ancestral strain in the vaccine and a higher prevalence of infection-induced immunity in the population overall during Omicron predominance,[73] which reduces the ability to measure VE. Data on vaccine effectiveness of bivalent boosters among pregnant people and infants are lacking at this time but are needed to inform COVID-19 vaccine policy recommendations. Data are also needed regarding the effectiveness among infants by timing of maternal vaccination, including for doses given before and during pregnancy.

SUMMARY

In conclusion, pregnant people are at increased risk of severe disease and adverse pregnancy outcomes from COVID-19, but initial COVID-19 vaccine clinical trials excluded pregnant people. Postauthorization studies have been important to fill evidence gaps regarding COVID-19 vaccine safety and effectiveness in pregnant people and infants, and lessons learned from the COVID-19 pandemic include the importance of including pregnant people in clinical trials when possible. Evidence has consistently demonstrated that COVID-19 mRNA vaccines are safe when given during pregnancy for both pregnant people and infants, and COVID-19 mRNA vaccines protect pregnant people and their infants who are too young to receive COVID-19 vaccines. Monovalent vaccine effectiveness was lower during Omicron predominance, and bivalent vaccines may improve protection against Omicron variants. Everyone, including people who are pregnant, breastfeeding, trying to get pregnant now, or might become pregnant in the future, should stay up to date with recommended COVID-19 vaccines and get the recommended bivalent booster, when eligible.

CLINICS CARE POINTS

- Everyone, including pregnant people, should stay up to date with recommended COVID-19 vaccines and get the recommended bivalent booster, when eligible.

DISCLAIMER

The findings and conclusions in this report are those of the authors and do not necessarily represent the official position of the Centers for Disease Control and Prevention. Mention of a product or company name is for identification purposes only and does not constitute endorsement by CDC.

DISCLOSURES

None of the authors have conflicts of interest.

FUNDING

This work was funded by the Centers for Disease Control and Prevention.

ACKNOWLEDGMENTS

The authors acknowledge that not every person who can become pregnant identifies as a woman. Although we try to use gender-neutral language as often as possible, much of the research available currently refers only to "women" when discussing the ability to become pregnant. When citing research, we refer to the language used in the study. In these cases, "woman" refers to someone who was assigned female at birth. For clarity in terminology, "maternal' is used to identify the person who is pregnant or post-partum throughout this article; the authors are aware that pregnancy is not equated with the decision to parent nor do all parents who give birth identify as mothers.

SUPPLEMENTARY DATA

Supplementary data related to this article can be found online at https://doi.org/10.1016/j.ogc.2023.02.003.

REFERENCES

1. Omer SB. Maternal Immunization. N Engl J Med 2017;376(13):1256–67.

2. Grohskopf LA, Blanton LH, Ferdinands JM, et al. Prevention and Control of Seasonal Influenza with Vaccines: Recommendations of the Advisory Committee on Immunization Practices - United States, 2022-23 Influenza Season. MMWR Recomm Rep (Morb Mortal Wkly Rep) 2022;71(1):1–28.

3. Centers for Disease Control and Prevention. Use of COVID-19 Vaccines in the United States: Interim Clinical Considerations. 2022. Available at: https://www.cdc.gov/vaccines/covid-19/clinical-considerations/covid-19-vaccines-us.html#:~:text=The%20CDC%20Interim%20Clinical%20Considerations%20are%20informed%20by,currently%20approved%20or%20authorized%20in%20the%20United%20States. Accessed October 19, 2022.

4. Liang JL, Tiwari T, Moro P, et al. Prevention of Pertussis, Tetanus, and Diphtheria with Vaccines in the United States: Recommendations of the Advisory Committee on Immunization Practices (ACIP). MMWR Recomm Rep (Morb Mortal Wkly Rep) 2018;67(2):1–44.

5. Allotey J, Stallings E, Bonet M, et al. Clinical manifestations, risk factors, and maternal and perinatal outcomes of coronavirus disease 2019 in pregnancy: living systematic review and meta-analysis. BMJ 2020;370:m3320. https://doi.org/10.1136/bmj.m3320.

6. Dooling K, Marin M, Wallace M, et al. The Advisory Committee on Immunization Practices' Updated Interim Recommendation for Allocation of COVID-19 Vaccine - United States, December 2020. MMWR Morb Mortal Wkly Rep 2021;69(5152):1657–60.

7. Dunkle LM, Kotloff KL, Gay CL, et al. Efficacy and Safety of NVX-CoV2373 in Adults in the United States and Mexico. N Engl J Med 2021;386(6):531–43.

8. El Sahly HM, Baden LR, Essink B, et al. Efficacy of the mRNA-1273 SARS-CoV-2 Vaccine at Completion of Blinded Phase. N Engl J Med 2021. https://doi.org/10.1056/NEJMoa2113017.

9. Polack FP, Thomas SJ, Kitchin N, et al. Safety and Efficacy of the BNT162b2 mRNA Covid-19 Vaccine. N Engl J Med 2020;383(27):2603–15.

10. Sadoff J, Gray G, Vandebosch A, et al. Safety and Efficacy of Single-Dose Ad26.COV2.S Vaccine against Covid-19. N Engl J Med 2021;384(23):2187–201.

11. Centers for Disease Control and Prevention. New CDC Data: COVID-19 Vaccination Safe for Pregnant People. Available at: https://www.cdc.gov/media/releases/2021/s0811-vaccine-safe-pregnant.html. Accessed October 26, 2022.

12. Atyeo CG, Shook LL, Brigida S, et al. Maternal immune response and placental antibody transfer after COVID-19 vaccination across trimester and platforms. Nat Commun 2022/06/28 2022;13(1):3571.

13. Prahl M, Golan Y, Cassidy AG, et al. Evaluation of transplacental transfer of mRNA vaccine products and functional antibodies during pregnancy and infancy. Nat Commun 2022/07/30 2022;13(1):4422.

14. Marks KJ, Whitaker M, Agathis NT, et al. Hospitalization of Infants and Children Aged 0-4 Years with Laboratory-Confirmed COVID-19 - COVID-NET, 14 States, March 2020-February 2022. MMWR Morb Mortal Wkly Rep 2022;71(11):429–36.

15. Hamid S, Woodworth K, Pham H, et al. COVID-19-Associated Hospitalizations Among U.S. Infants Aged <6 Months - COVID-NET, 13 States, June 2021-August 2022. MMWR Morb Mortal Wkly Rep 2022;71(45):1442–8.

16. Delahoy MJ, Ujamaa D, Taylor CA, et al. Comparison of influenza and COVID-19-associated hospitalizations among children < 18 years old in the United States-FluSurv-NET (October-April 2017-2021) and COVID-NET (October 2020-September 2021). Clin Infect Dis 2022. https://doi.org/10.1093/cid/ciac388.

17. Chaves SS, Perez A, Farley MM, et al. The burden of influenza hospitalizations in infants from 2003 to 2012, United States. Pediatr Infect Dis J. Sep 2014;33(9):912–9.

18. Badell ML, Dude CM, Rasmussen SA, et al. Covid-19 vaccination in pregnancy. BMJ 2022;378:e069741.

19. Prasad S, Kalafat E, Blakeway H, et al. Systematic review and meta-analysis of the effectiveness and perinatal outcomes of COVID-19 vaccination in pregnancy. Nat Commun 2022;13(1):2414.

20. Watanabe A, Yasuhara J, Iwagami M, et al. Peripartum Outcomes Associated With COVID-19 Vaccination During Pregnancy: A Systematic Review and Meta-analysis. JAMA Pediatr 2022.

21. Rosenblum HG, Wallace M, Godfrey M, et al. Interim Recommendations from the Advisory Committee on Immunization Practices for the Use of Bivalent Booster Doses of COVID-19 Vaccines - United States, October 2022. MMWR Morb Mortal Wkly Rep 2022;71(45):1436–41.

22. Centers for Disease Control and Prevention. COVID-19 Vaccination Coverage and Vaccine Confidence Among Adults: COVIDVaxView. Available at: https://www.cdc.gov/vaccines/imz-managers/coverage/covidvaxview/interactive/adults.html. Accessed November 14, 2022.

23. Rasmussen SA, Kelley CF, Horton JP, et al. Coronavirus Disease 2019 (COVID-19) Vaccines and Pregnancy: What Obstetricians Need to Know. Obstet Gynecol 2021;137(3):408–14.

24. Food and Drug Administration VaRBPAC. FDA briefing document: Moderna COVID-19 Vaccine; Vaccines and related biological products Advisory committee meeting December. 2020. https://www.fda.gov/media/144434/download.

25. Food and Drug Administration VaRBPAC, FDA briefing document: Pfizer-BioNTech COVID-19 Vaccine: Vaccines and Related Biological Products Advisory Committee meeting December 10, 2020, Available at: https://www.fda.gov/media/144245/download, 2020. Accessed November 15, 2022.

26. Shimabukuro TT, Kim SY, Myers TR, et al. Preliminary Findings of mRNA Covid-19 Vaccine Safety in Pregnant Persons. N Engl J Med 2021;384(24):2273–82.

27. Favre G, Maisonneuve E, Pomar L, et al. COVID-19 mRNA vaccine in pregnancy: Results of the Swiss COVI-PREG registry, an observational prospective cohort study. Lancet Reg Health Eur. Jul 2022;18:100410.

28. Bookstein Peretz S, Regev N, Novick L, et al. Short-term outcome of pregnant women vaccinated with BNT162b2 mRNA COVID-19 vaccine. Ultrasound Obstet Gynecol 2021;58(3):450–6.

29. Sadarangani M, Soe P, Shulha HP, et al. Safety of COVID-19 vaccines in pregnancy: a Canadian National Vaccine Safety (CANVAS) network cohort study. Lancet Infect Dis. Aug 2022;11:11. https://doi.org/10.1016/S1473-3099(22)00426-1.

30. DeSilva M, Haapala J, Vazquez-Benitez G, et al. Evaluation of Acute Adverse Events after Covid-19 Vaccination during Pregnancy. N Engl J Med 2022; 387(2):187–9.

31. Moro PL, Olson CK, Clark E, et al. Post-authorization surveillance of adverse events following COVID-19 vaccines in pregnant persons in the vaccine adverse event reporting system (VAERS), 2020 - 2021. Vaccine 2022;40(24):3389–94.

32. Moro PL, Olson CK, Zhang B, et al. Safety of Booster Doses of Coronavirus Disease 2019 (COVID-19) Vaccine in Pregnancy in the Vaccine Adverse Event Reporting System. Obstet Gynecol 2022;140(3):421–7.

33. Mukherjee S, Velez Edwards DR, Baird DD, et al. Risk of miscarriage among black women and white women in a U.S. Prospective Cohort Study. Am J Epidemiol 2013;177(11):1271–8.

34. Goldhaber MK, Fireman BH. The fetal life table revisited: spontaneous abortion rates in three Kaiser Permanente cohorts. Epidemiology 1991;2(1):33–9.

35. Xu R, Luo Y, Chambers C. Assessing the effect of vaccine on spontaneous abortion using time-dependent covariates Cox models. Pharmacoepidemiol Drug Saf 2012;21(8):844–50.

36. Zauche LH, Wallace B, Smoots AN, et al. Receipt of mRNA Covid-19 Vaccines and Risk of Spontaneous Abortion. N Engl J Med 2021;385(16):1533–5.

37. Citu IM, Citu C, Gorun F, et al. The Risk of Spontaneous Abortion Does Not Increase Following First Trimester mRNA COVID-19 Vaccination. J Clin Med 2022;11(6):18.

38. Kharbanda EO, Haapala J, DeSilva M, et al. Spontaneous Abortion Following COVID-19 Vaccination During Pregnancy. JAMA 2021;326(16):1629–31.

39. Magnus MC, Gjessing HK, Eide HN, et al. Covid-19 Vaccination during Pregnancy and First-Trimester Miscarriage. N Engl J Med 2021;385(21):2008–10.

40. Gregory ECW VC, Hoyert DL. Fetal mortality: United States, 2020. Natl Vital Stat Rep 2022;71.

41. DeSisto CL, Wallace B, Simeone RM, et al. Risk for Stillbirth Among Women With and Without COVID-19 at Delivery Hospitalization - United States, March 2020-September 2021. MMWR Morb Mortal Wkly Rep 2021;70(47):1640–5.

42. Magnus MC, Ortqvist AK, Dahlqwist E, et al. Association of SARS-CoV-2 Vaccination During Pregnancy With Pregnancy Outcomes. JAMA 2022;327(15):1469–77.

43. Hui L, Marzan MB, Rolnik DL, et al. Reductions in stillbirths and preterm birth in COVID-19 vaccinated women: a multi-center cohort study of vaccination uptake and perinatal outcomes. Am J Obstet Gynecol 2022. https://doi.org/10.1016/j.ajog.2022.10.040.

44. Dick A, Rosenbloom JI, Gutman-Ido E, et al. Safety of SARS-CoV-2 vaccination during pregnancy- obstetric outcomes from a large cohort study. BMC Pregnancy Childbirth 2022;22(1):166.

45. Peretz-Machluf R, Hirsh-Yechezkel G, Zaslavsky-Paltiel I, et al. Obstetric and Neonatal Outcomes following COVID-19 Vaccination in Pregnancy. J Clin Med 2022;11(9):30.

46. Theiler RN, Wick M, Mehta R, et al. Pregnancy and birth outcomes after SARS-CoV-2 vaccination in pregnancy. Am J Obstet Gynecol MFM 2021;3(6):100467.

47. Wainstock T, Yoles I, Sergienko R, et al. Prenatal maternal COVID-19 vaccination and pregnancy outcomes. Vaccine 2021;39(41):6037–40.

48. Bleicher I, Kadour-Peero E, Sagi-Dain L, et al. Early exploration of COVID-19 vaccination safety and effectiveness during pregnancy: interim descriptive data from a prospective observational study. Vaccine 2021;39(44):6535–8.

49. Blakeway H, Prasad S, Kalafat E, et al. COVID-19 vaccination during pregnancy: coverage and safety. Am J Obstet Gynecol 2022;226(2):236 e1–e236 e14.

50. Fell DB, Dhinsa T, Alton GD, et al. Association of COVID-19 Vaccination in Pregnancy With Adverse Peripartum Outcomes. JAMA 2022;327(15):1478–87.

51. Rottenstreich M, Sela HY, Rotem R, et al. Covid-19 vaccination during the third trimester of pregnancy: rate of vaccination and maternal and neonatal outcomes, a multicentre retrospective cohort study. BJOG 2022;129(2):248–55.

52. Di Girolamo R, Khalil A, Alameddine S, et al. Placental histopathology after SARS-CoV-2 infection in pregnancy: a systematic review and meta-analysis. Am J Obstet Gynecol MFM 2021;3(6):100468.

53. Shanes ED, Otero S, Mithal LB, et al. Severe Acute Respiratory Syndrome Coronavirus 2 (SARS-CoV-2) Vaccination in Pregnancy: Measures of Immunity and Placental Histopathology. Obstet Gynecol 2021;138(2):281–3.

54. Boelig RC, Aghai ZH, Chaudhury S, et al. Impact of COVID-19 disease and COVID-19 vaccination on maternal or fetal inflammatory response, placental pathology, and perinatal outcomes. Am J Obstet Gynecol 2022;227(4):652–6.

55. Neelam V, Reeves EL, Woodworth KR, et al. Pregnancy and infant outcomes by trimester of SARS-CoV-2 infection in pregnancy–SET-NET, 22 jurisdictions. Birth Defects Research 2020. https://doi.org/10.1002/bdr2.2081.

56. Lipkind HS, Vazquez-Benitez G, DeSilva M, et al. Receipt of COVID-19 Vaccine During Pregnancy and Preterm or Small-for-Gestational-Age at Birth - Eight Integrated Health Care Organizations, United States, December 15, 2020-July 22, 2021. MMWR Morb Mortal Wkly Rep 7 2022;71(1):26–30.

57. Goldshtein I, Steinberg DM, Kuint J, et al. Association of BNT162b2 COVID-19 Vaccination During Pregnancy With Neonatal and Early Infant Outcomes. JAMA Pediatr 2022;176(5):470–7.

58. Stock SJ, Carruthers J, Calvert C, et al. SARS-CoV-2 infection and COVID-19 vaccination rates in pregnant women in Scotland. Nat Med 2022;28(3):504–12.

59. Ruderman RS, Mormol J, Trawick E, et al. Association of COVID-19 Vaccination During Early Pregnancy With Risk of Congenital Fetal Anomalies. JAMA Pediatr 2022;176(7):717–9.

60. Mai CT, Isenburg JL, Canfield MA, et al. National population-based estimates for major birth defects, 2010–2014. Birth Defects Research 2019;111(18):1420–35.

61. Goldshtein I, Nevo D, Steinberg DM, et al. Association Between BNT162b2 Vaccination and Incidence of SARS-CoV-2 Infection in Pregnant Women. JAMA 2021;326(8):728–35.

62. Dagan N, Barda N, Biron-Shental T, et al. Effectiveness of the BNT162b2 mRNA COVID-19 vaccine in pregnancy. Nat Med 2021/10/01 2021;27(10):1693–5.

63. Butt AA, Chemaitelly H, Al Khal A, et al. SARS-CoV-2 vaccine effectiveness in preventing confirmed infection in pregnant women. J Clin Invest 2021;131(23).

64. Dagan N, Barda N, Kepten E, et al. BNT162b2 mRNA Covid-19 Vaccine in a Nationwide Mass Vaccination Setting. N Engl J Med 2021;384(15):1412–23.
65. Abu-Raddad LJ, Chemaitelly H, Butt AA. Effectiveness of the BNT162b2 Covid-19 Vaccine against the B.1.1.7 and B.1.351 Variants. N Engl J Med 2021; 385(2):187–9.
66. Schrag SJ, Verani JR, Dixon BE, et al. Estimation of COVID-19 mRNA Vaccine Effectiveness Against Medically Attended COVID-19 in Pregnancy During Periods of Delta and Omicron Variant Predominance in the United States. JAMA Netw Open 2022;5(9):e2233273.
67. Guedalia J, Lipschuetz M, Calderon-Margalit R, et al. Effectiveness of a third BNT162b2 mRNA COVID-19 vaccination during pregnancy: a national observational study in Israel. Nat Commun 2022;13:6961. https://doi.org/10.1038/s41467-022-34605-x.
68. Magnus MC, Håberg SE, Carlsen EØ, et al. Pregnancy status at the time of COVID-19 vaccination and incidence of SARS-CoV-2 infection. Clin Infect Dis 2022. https://doi.org/10.1093/cid/ciac739.
69. Halasa NB, Olson SM, Staat MA, et al. Effectiveness of Maternal Vaccination with mRNA COVID-19 Vaccine During Pregnancy Against COVID-19-Associated Hospitalization in Infants Aged <6 Months - 17 States, July 2021-January 2022. MMWR Morb Mortal Wkly Rep 2022;71(7):264–70.
70. Halasa NB, Olson SM, Staat MA, et al. Maternal Vaccination and Risk of Hospitalization for Covid-19 among Infants. N Engl J Med 2022;387(2):109–19.
71. Carlsen EO, Magnus MC, Oakley L, et al. Association of COVID-19 Vaccination During Pregnancy With Incidence of SARS-CoV-2 Infection in Infants. JAMA Intern Med 2022;182(8):825–31.
72. Zerbo O, Ray GT, Fireman B, et al. Maternal SARS-CoV-2 Vaccination and Infant Protection Against SARS-CoV-2 During the First Six Months of Life. Nat Commun 2023;14(894). https://doi.org/10.1038/s41467-023-36547-4.
73. Clarke KEN, Jones JM, Deng Y, et al. Seroprevalence of Infection-Induced SARS-CoV-2 Antibodies - United States, September 2021-February 2022. MMWR Morb Mortal Wkly Rep 2022;71(17):606–8.

An Update on Gonorrhea and Chlamydia

Karley Dutra, MD*, Gweneth Lazenby, MD, MSCP

KEYWORDS

• Gonorrhea • Chlamydia • Cervicitis • STD screening

KEY POINTS

- Chlamydia and gonorrhea are the two most common notifiable sexually transmitted infections in the United States, with significant long-term health impacts including pelvic inflammatory disease (PID), infertility, and ectopic pregnancy.
- Preferred treatment of these infections continues to evolve with the most recent Centers for Disease Control and Prevention (CDC) guidelines from 2021 recommending doxycycline 100 mg BID for 7 days for treatment of chlamydia in non-pregnant persons due to superior cure of rectal infections.
- Due to potential drug resistance, higher doses of ceftriaxone intramuscularly are the preferred treatment of gonorrhea infections and dual therapy is no longer recommended.
- Future research should determine effective strategies for the prevention of chlamydia and gonorrhea transmission, such as pre- or post-exposure prophylaxis.

INTRODUCTION

Gonorrhea and chlamydia infections are the two most common notifiable sexually transmitted infections in the United States. Both have the potential for significant sequelae for the female reproductive tract including pelvic inflammatory disease (PID), ectopic pregnancy, and infertility. To prevent these morbid conditions, it is important to screen persons at risk and promptly diagnose and treat gonorrhea and chlamydia infections.

Chlamydia is caused by infection with the obligate intracellular bacterium *chlamydia trachomatis* (*Chlamydia trachomatis*). *C Trachomatis* is divided into three biovars which each causing clinically distinct disease states. Each biovar of *C trachomatis* can be subdivided into serovars, with serovars D-K causing urogenital and conjunctival infections and serovars L1-L3 causing the genital infection lymphogranuloma venereum (LGV). The last biovar consists of serovars A, B, and C which causes trachoma. LGV infection presents as a painless genital ulcer with associated inguinal

Department of Obstetrics and Gynecology, Medical University of South Carolina, 96 Jonathan Lucas Street, Charleston, SC 29425, USA
* Corresponding author.
E-mail address: karleydutra@gmail.com

Obstet Gynecol Clin N Am 50 (2023) 299–310
https://doi.org/10.1016/j.ogc.2023.02.004
0889-8545/23/© 2023 Elsevier Inc. All rights reserved.

lymphadenopathy. Additionally, LVG can cause proctocolitis by gaining entry to the rectum via breaks in the skin or through epithelial cells of the genital tract or rectum. In the female genital tract, C trachomatis serovars D-K target squamocolumnar epithelial cells of the endocervix and upper genital tract leading to a mucopurulent drainage in some patients. Approximately, 70% of cis women will be asymptomatic.[1,2]

Neisseria gonorrhoeae, a gram-negative coccobacillus, infects the columnar cells of the cervix resulting in mucopurulent cervicitis. Most women with urogenital gonorrhea infection are asymptomatic, but symptoms of cervicitis may include purulent vaginal discharge and abnormal uterine bleeding.[1,2]

Chlamydia trachomatis is the most common notifiable sexually transmitted infection in the United States. Chlamydia infections are most often diagnosed in persons younger than 25.[3] Preliminary national surveillance data from 2021 suggest that the number of chlamydia cases in the United States have been steadily rising after a brief decline in 2019 and 2020.[4] Public health officials suggest that the decline in the reported number of chlamydia diagnoses was more likely related to restricted access to screening during the coronavirus disease 2019 (COVID-19) pandemic rather than fewer infections. Continued surveillance over the next several years should elucidate the extent to which the pandemic impacted the number of chlamydia cases in 2021.[5]

Gonorrhea is the second most common notifiable sexually transmitted infection in the United States. The number of reported gonorrhea cases in the United States has increased by more than 100% since 2009. Dissimilar to chlamydia, the COVID-19 pandemic did not affect the number of reported cases.[3] It is difficult to draw conclusions as to why cases of gonorrhea increased during the COVID pandemic whereas cases of chlamydia decreased, but surveillance data collected in the following years should provide clarity.

Clinical Impact

Persistent lower genital tract infections with chlamydia and gonorrhea can ascend into the upper female genital tract, leading to pelvic inflammatory disease (PID). PID is associated with long-term sequelae including ectopic pregnancy and tubal factor infertility.[6–9] Multiple studies have reported an association between chlamydia infection and these sequelae, including a retrospective observational study of 857,324 cis women over 14 years (2000–2013).[6–8,10] Compared with persons who screened negative, chlamydia diagnosis was associated with a 135% increased risk of PID, 90% increased risk of ectopic pregnancy, and 70% increased risk of infertility.[10] Compared with chlamydia, gonorrhea has been associated with more severe symptoms of PID, including purulent cervicitis and fevers, and higher rates of hospitalization.[7,11]

Extragenital chlamydia and gonorrhea can occur in the oropharynx, rectum, and eyes. The reported prevalence of extragenital infections varies in cis women by site and organism. Oropharyngeal infections range from 0% to 29.6% (median 2.1%, gonorrhea) and 0.2% to 3.2% (median 1.7%, chlamydia). Rectal infections range from 0.6% to 35.8% (median 1.9%, gonorrhea) and 2.0% to 77.3% (median 8.7%, chlamydia). A significant portion of persons with rectal infections do not report receptive anal sex.[12] Most extragenital chlamydial infections are asymptomatic. Infrequently infected persons can develop asymmetric mono- or oligoarthritis (reactive arthritis) after symptomatic urogenital chlamydia infection.[9,13] Rarely, N gonorrhoeae can cause disseminated gonococcal infection presenting as asymmetric polyarthralgia, septic arthritis, tenosynovitis, or petechial skin lesions.

Antenatal infection with either chlamydia or gonorrhea has been associated with adverse pregnancy and neonatal outcomes. Untreated infection is associated with increased risks of premature rupture of membranes, low birth weight infants, and preterm delivery.[14,15] Additionally, untreated chlamydial infection during pregnancy has been associated with an increased risk of pregnancy loss including early miscarriage and intrauterine fetal demise.[16,17] There is limited evidence to suggest treatment of chlamydia and gonorrhea infection during pregnancy may reduce the risk of adverse pregnancy outcomes.[18] Newborns exposed to chlamydia or gonorrhea during delivery can develop conjunctivitis from either or chlamydial pneumonia. Treatment significantly reduces the percentage of newborns who develop chlamydia conjunctivitis: 30% to 50% of infants born to untreated persons and less than 1% of infants born to treated persons.[9,15,19,20]

Evaluation

Annual screening for both urogenital gonorrhea and chlamydia is recommended for all sexually active cis women <25 years old, and those older than 25 years old who are at increased risk for infection. Extragenital chlamydia and gonorrhea screening can be considered based on risk factors and area of residence. Recent evidence suggests that routine extragenital screening should be considered given reported sexual behavior often does not align wtih positivity at extragenital sites.[12,21] Risk factors for chlamydia and gonorrhea infection include multiple or new sexual partners, sexual partners with known sexually transmitted infections (STIs), sexual partners with other concurrent partners, inconsistent condom use, or the exchange of sex for money or drugs. Screening is recommended for incarcerated cis women younger than 35 years old given the high prevalence of infection among these persons.[22] Chlamydia screening is recommended at the first prenatal visit in persons < 25 years old. Persons at increased risk for infection should be screened again in the third trimester. Pregnant people at risk or residing in high-prevalence areas should also be screened for gonorrhea.

Early screening and treatment of chlamydial infection moderately reduce the number of PID cases compared with unscreened populations.[23–25] To date, no studies have directly evaluated the effectiveness of gonorrhea screening in the reduction of PID cases or other sequela of untreated infection. More frequent screening may be indicated in persons with risk factors for infection, and an emphasis should be placed on partner testing and treatment to prevent reinfection.

Urogenital chlamydia and gonorrhea can be diagnosed using vaginal or endocervical swabs or first-void urine samples. Nucleic acid amplification tests (NAAT) from vaginal swabs have the highest sensitivity and specificity for both chlamydia and gonorrhea diagnoses. Sensitivity and specificity of NAATs are similar for patient and provider-collected vaginal swabs. Self-collection is associated with high patient satisfaction, making this a reasonably preferred approach if a pelvic exam is not otherwise indicated.[26,27] Both chlamydia and gonorrhea NAATs can be collected from liquid-based cervical cytology, although this is less sensitive than vaginal swabs and urine specimens. NAATs are preferred to culture for gonorrhea testing due to higher sensitivity and specificity, but culture is indicated if there is suspected or confirmed treatment failure to determine antimicrobial susceptibilities. Testing for rectal and oropharyngeal gonorrhea and chlamydia is preferentially done using NAATs from swabs. Point-of-care NAATs testing is Food and Drug Administration (FDA)-approved for all swab collections for both chlamydia and gonorrhea and offers the benefit of prompt diagnosis and treatment.[28,29]

Therapeutic Options

Prompt diagnosis and treatment are important to prevent the long-term sequelae of chlamydia and gonorrhea infections, to prevent the continued transmission of these STIs, and to prevent adverse pregnancy and neonatal outcomes.

Extragenital chlamydial infection is more frequent than expected based on reported sexual practices. Doxycycline is more efficacious than azithromycin in treating rectal chlamydia among men who have sex with men (MSM) and cis women.[30,31] In one randomized controlled trial, the microbiological cure was 78.5% for azithromycin-treated rectal chlamydia infections compared with 95.5% in doxycycline-treated rectal infections in cis women, which is similar to the cure rates seen among the MSM population.[31,32] For rectal chlamydia infection, doxycycline has superior efficacy compared with azithromycin given unrecognized and inadequately treated rectal chlamydia infection in cis women can lead to recurrent urogenital infection via autoinoculation. The 2021 Center for Disease Control and Prevention Sexually Transmitted Guidelines recommend adolescents and adults should be preferentially treated with doxycycline 100 mg by mouth twice daily for 7 days. Azithromycin remains an alternative treatment of adolescents and adults, and the recommended treatment in pregnancy due to the risk of fetal tooth discoloration with doxycycline use in pregnancy.[29]

Neisseria species possess mechanisms such as plasmids that allow for the transfer of genetic material and deoxyribonucleic acid (DNA) that confer antimicrobial resistance. Gonorrhea treatment strategies have been and continue to be impacted by the organism's ability to develop antimicrobial resistance. The CDC Gonococcal Isolate Surveillance Project (GISP) monitors antimicrobial resistance to inform treatment recommendations for gonococcal infections. In the early 2000s, increasing resistance to fluoroquinolones resulted in limited antimicrobial options and cephalosporins are the last primary drug class available for treatment. Co-treatment with azithromycin or doxycycline and cephalosporin was previously recommended to reduce the development of antimicrobial resistance in gonorrhea.[33] Doxycycline is no longer recommended for dual treatment due to high resistance levels reported in GISP.[28] According to the GISP isolates from 2015 to 2019, the percentage of isolates with azithromycin mean inhibitory concentrations (MICs) ≥ 2.0 µg/mL had increased from 2.6% in 2015% to 5.1% in 2019. The percentage of isolates in GISP demonstrating reduced susceptibility to ceftriaxone remains low (<0.1% with MICs ≥ 0.5 µg/mL). Due to MIC creep for macrolide antimicrobials, the current strategy is to use higher doses of cephalosporins rather than give dual treatment.[34] Given the increase in gonococcal antimicrobial resistance, a concern for lower efficacy in the treatment of urogenital and rectal chlamydia, and efforts to improve antimicrobial stewardship, azithromycin is no longer a preferred therapy for gonorrhea infection.[35]

Based on existing evidence and trends in antimicrobial resistance, the preferred treatment of adults and adolescents with uncomplicated gonococcal infection of the urogenital tract, rectum, or oropharynx is ceftriaxone 500 mg intramuscularly (IM) for a single dose if the patient weighs less than 150 kg and ceftriaxone 1 g IM for a single dose if the patient weighs more than 150 kg.[28] No reliable treatment alternative is available for oropharyngeal gonorrhea. Providers should consult a local infectious disease specialist for patients who have a cephalosporin allergy or other contraindications to treatment with ceftriaxone. Below is **Table 1** summarizing the recommended treatments of both gonorrhea and chlamydia in adults and adolescents.

Partner Therapy

Prompt diagnosis and treatment of persons with gonorrhea and/or chlamydia infections and partner therapy are recommended strategies to reduce new cases of these sexually transmitted infections in the United States. Expedited partner therapy (EPT) refers to treatment prescribed to partners of persons being treated for sexually transmitted infection(s) without the need for an individual evaluation of infection.[36] EPT is currently approved in 46 states and is potentially allowable in the remaining 4 states.[37]

Table 1
Recommended and alternative treatments for chlamydia and gonorrhea

	Recommended Treatment	Alternative Treatment	Recommended Treatment in Pregnancy
Chlamydia trachomatis	Doxycycline 100 mg PO BID for 7 d	Azithromycin 1 g PO for a single dose Or Levofloxacin 500 mg PO daily for 7 d	Azithromycin 1 g PO for a single dose
Neisseria gonorrhea	Ceftriaxone 500 mg IM for a single dose if < 150 kg Ceftriaxone 1 g IM for a single dose if ≥ 150 kg	Cephalosporin allergy Gentamycin 240 mg IM for a single dose + Azithromycin 2 g PO for a single dose[a] Ceftriaxone not available Cefixime 800 mg PO for a single dose[a]	Ceftriaxone 500 mg IM for a single dose if < 150 kg Ceftriaxone 1 g IM for a single dose if ≥ 150 kg

[a] No reliable alternative treatment exists for the treatment of oropharyngeal gonorrhea infection and providers should contact an infectious disease specialist for assistance in patients who cannot receive ceftriaxone.

EPT is a safe and effective strategy for treating and preventing new and recurrent sexually transmitted infections.[38,39] Additionally, EPT has the potential to reduce health disparities among low-income patients and in communities of color by reducing stigma and by providing treatment to those with limited access to health care.[40] EPT is perceived as convenient and reasonable by adolescents, who are at increased risk for sexually transmitted infections.[41] Among adults being treated for chlamydia and gonorrhea, EPT has been shown to be acceptable and perceived to reduce rates of sexually transmitted infections.[42,43]

Follow-up After Treatment

To prevent transmission of gonorrhea and chlamydia to susceptible partner(s), persons diagnosed and receiving treatment of these infections should be counseled to abstain from unprotected intercourse for 7 days after a single-dose treatment. If treated with a 7-day course of antibiotics, unprotected intercourse should be avoided until the course of treatment is complete and symptoms, if present, have resolved. To prevent reinfection, all partners should be treated before resumption of unprotected intercourse, either by EPT (described above) or after evaluation by a health care provider.

Test of Cure

A test of cure (TOC) refers to repeat testing following treatment to ensure clearance of a sexually transmitted infection. NAATs, which are the most frequently used diagnostic tests for gonorrhea and chlamydia, are highly sensitive and specific. NAATs can detect any genetic material regardless of its biologic activity. Treated persons may continue to have a positive NAATs test for gonorrhea or chlamydia for a period of 3 to 4 weeks. There is currently no consensus on when a TOC should be collected to reliably expect a negative NAATs after treatment regardless of the site of infection (ie, urogenital, rectal, or oropharyngeal). The cost-effectiveness of the TOC strategy may be limited due to a low likelihood of positive tests after adequate treatment.[44–46]

For adults and adolescents, TOC is recommended for those with oropharyngeal gonorrhea infection. Oropharyngeal gonorrhea is more challenging to treat due to poor penetration of antibiotics into the pharynx leading to overall lower tissue drug levels. This can lead to preferential selection of gonococcal isolates with elevated MICs and therefore possible treatment failure. Current guidelines recommend performing a TOC with NAATs 7 to 14 days after initial treatment with previous studies demonstrating a higher likelihood of false positives at day 7 compared with days 10 to 14 due to residual non-biologically active genetic material.[47,48] Preferentially, TOC for oropharyngeal gonorrhea infection should be collected ≥ 10 days following treatment. NAAT has been demonstrated to be more sensitive when compared with culture for the detection of oropharyngeal gonorrhea.[49,50] NAAT has been used in previous studies evaluating the effectiveness of TOC for oropharyngeal gonorrhea infection and remains the recommended test.[47] If there is a concern for gonococcal antimicrobial resistance, then culture should be performed to determine antimicrobial susceptibilities.

TOC is recommended in pregnancy to minimize the potential risks to both the mother and fetus of untreated chlamydia and/or gonorrhea infection. In a study following both pregnant and non-pregnant women diagnosed with vaginal chlamydial infection and treated with single-dose azithromycin, the median time to a negative NAAT for all participants was 12 days, and by day 29 post-treatment, 100% of participants who presented on time for specimen submission had negative chlamydia NAAT tests. Additionally, 94% of pregnant participants and 96% of non-pregnant participants had negative testing by day 20 post-treatment.[51] These findings suggest and are aligned with current CDC STD screening guidelines, that for pregnant women diagnosed with urogenital chlamydia, a TOC should not be performed sooner than 3 to 4 weeks post-treatment.

A TOC for gonorrhea or chlamydia is therefore indicated for the following individuals.

- Adolescents or adults with oropharyngeal gonorrhea infection ≥ 10 days after treatment to minimize the risk of false positive NAATs
- Pregnant persons with urogenital chlamydia and/or gonorrhea infection 3 to 4 weeks after treatment completed

A TOC for gonorrhea or chlamydia is not recommended for the following individuals.

- Non-pregnant persons with urogenital or rectal gonorrhea infection
- Non-pregnant persons with urogenital, rectal, or oropharyngeal chlamydial infection

TOC is not indicated in persons prescribed an alternative treatment regimen for chlamydia or gonorrhea. Current guidelines recommend retesting at 3 months in the above individuals to ensure reinfection has not occurred. Repeat testing may be indicated sooner in patients with persistent symptoms, concern for reinfection, or an inability to complete the entire treatment as prescribed. Of note, retesting at 3 months is not considered to be a TOC as it is performed to evaluate for reinfection remote from the initial infection.

Table 2 below is a summary of recommended testing guidelines after initial infection with gonorrhea or chlamydia in both pregnant and non-pregnant adults.

PREVENTION AND FUTURE DIRECTIONS

Strategies for prevention of gonorrhea and chlamydia infection are currently prompt diagnosis and treatment, and EPT. Post-exposure prophylaxis (PEP) with oral

Table 2
Guideline for performing TOC for chlamydia and gonorrhea

Population	Infection and Site	TOC in 7–14 d	TOC in 4 wks	Retest in 3 mo	Retest Within 1 y
Non-pregnant adults	Urogenital, rectal, oropharyngeal chlamydia	Not Recommended	Not Recommended	Recommended	Recommended if not tested at 3 mo
Pregnant adults	Urogenital, rectal, oropharyngeal chlamydia	Not Recommended	Recommended	Recommended	Recommend repeat testing again in the third trimester
Non-pregnant adults	Urogenital, rectal gonorrhea	Not Recommended	Not Recommended	Recommended	Recommended if not tested at 3 mo
Pregnant adults	Urogenital, rectal gonorrhea	Not Recommended	Recommended	Recommended	Recommend repeat testing again in the third trimester
All adolescents and adults	Oropharyngeal gonorrhea	Recommended	Not Recommended	Recommended	Recommended if not tested at 3 mo

doxycycline is a potential future strategy with limited evidence in studies of MSM and transgender women (TGW). In a randomized open-label study including 554 individuals prescribed either pre-exposure prophylaxis for HIV prevention or anti-retroviral therapy for treatment of HIV, doxycycline 200 mg one time within 72 hours of unprotected intercourse resulted in a significant reduction in the number of new STI diagnoses. Those who received doxycycline PEP did not have any significant adverse events associated with PEP.[52]

Doxycycline has been associated with adverse side effects, including gastrointestinal upset, phototoxicity, and esophageal ulceration, and more studies are needed to evaluate the incidence and severity of adverse outcomes among people taking doxycycline PEP.[53] Future studies are needed to further delineate the populations for whom this intervention would be effective including cis women and transmen.

SUMMARY

Chlamydia and gonorrhea are the two most common notifiable sexually transmitted infections according to the CDC, with a significant disease among persons 24 years old and younger. Screening remains an important strategy to limit the transmission of both infections. Long-term health sequela for cis women include higher rates of PID, ectopic pregnancy, and tubal factor infertility. Additionally, infection in pregnancy can lead to premature rupture of membranes, preterm delivery, low birth weight, and neonatal infections including conjunctivitis and pneumonia.

Encouraging safe sex practices, rapid diagnosis, treatment, and EPT are currently the main strategies to prevent transmission of chlamydia and gonorrhea. Looking ahead, we anticipate strategies such as PEP may be beneficial to prevent transmission of these infections. More research is needed to determine the efficacy and safety, along with appropriate target populations, for a strategy like doxycycline PEP.

CLINICS CARE POINTS

- Chlamydia and gonorrhea are the two most common notifiable sexually transmitted diseases in the United States and untreated infection can be associated with PID, infertility, and ectopic pregnancy.

- Gonorrhea and chlamydia infections in pregnancy are associated with an increased risk of preterm premature rupture of membranes (PPROM), low birth weight infants, and preterm delivery. There are conflicting data regarding if treatment leads to improved neonatal outcomes, but current guidelines recommend routine screening, treatment, and TOC to mitigate any adverse effects of these infections in pregnancy.

- Annual screening for urogenital chlamydia and gonorrhea is recommended for cis women < 25 years of age due to the increased rates of infection among this population. Additional screening is recommended for cis women older than 25 if they have risk factors for STDs.

- Extragenital screening (oropharyngeal, rectal) is not currently routinely recommended and should be considered for persons reporting oral and/or anal sex.

- The preferred method of testing for both gonorrhea and chlamydia is NAATs due to superior sensitivity and specificity.

- The recommended treatment of chlamydia in non-pregnant persons is doxycycline 100 mg by mouth twice a day for 7 days. Azithromycin 1000 mg by mouth once remains the recommended treatment in pregnancy.

- Ceftriaxone 500 mg intramuscularly is the preferred treatment of gonorrhea in all persons.

- EPT is a safe and patient-acceptable strategy to reduce transmission of chlamydia and gonorrhea.
- TOC is recommended 3 to 4 weeks after treatment of pregnant persons with either gonorrhea and/or chlamydia.
- Doxycycline PEP is effective in preventing recurrent STIs among MSM and TGW with more studies needed to determine the safety and efficacy among other populations.

DISCLOSURES

No relevant disclosures.

REFERENCES

1. Loscalzo J, Fauci AS, Kasper DL, et al. Harrison's principles of internal medicine. 21st edition. New York: McGraw Hill; 2022.
2. Ryan KJ. Sherris & Ryan's medical microbiology. 8th edition. New York: McGraw Hill; 2022.
3. Division of STD Prevention NCfH. Viral Hepatitis, STD, and TB Prevention. National Overview of STDs, 2020. Secondary National Overview of STDs, 2020. 2022. https://www.cdc.gov/std/statistics/2020/overview.htm.
4. Division of STD Prevention NCfH. Viral Hepatitis, STD, and TB Prevention. Preliminary 2021 STD Survellience Data. Secondary Preliminary 2021 STD Survellience Data. 2022. Available at: https://www.cdc.gov/std/statistics/2021/default.htm.
5. Division of STD Prevention NCfH. Viral Hepatitis, STD, and TB Prevention. Impact of COVID-19 on STDs. Secondary Impact of COVID-19 on STDs. 2022. Available at: https://www.cdc.gov/std/statistics/2020/impact.htm.
6. Haggerty CL, Gottlieb SL, Taylor BD, et al. Risk of sequelae after Chlamydia trachomatis genital infection in women. J Infect Dis 2010;201(Suppl 2):S134–55.
7. Reekie J, Donovan B, Guy R, et al. Risk of Pelvic Inflammatory Disease in Relation to Chlamydia and Gonorrhea Testing, Repeat Testing, and Positivity: A Population-Based Cohort Study. Clin Infect Dis 2018;66(3):437–43.
8. Davies B, Turner KME, Frølund M, et al. Risk of reproductive complications following chlamydia testing: a population-based retrospective cohort study in Denmark. Lancet Infect Dis 2016;16(9):1057–64.
9. Tuddenham S, Hamill MM, Ghanem KG. Diagnosis and Treatment of Sexually Transmitted Infections: A Review. JAMA 2022;327(2):161–72.
10. den Heijer CDJ, Hoebe CJPA, Driessen JHM, et al. Chlamydia trachomatis and the Risk of Pelvic Inflammatory Disease, Ectopic Pregnancy, and Female Infertility: A Retrospective Cohort Study Among Primary Care Patients. Clin Infect Dis 2019;69(9):1517–25.
11. Short VL, Totten PA, Ness RB, et al. Clinical presentation of Mycoplasma genitalium Infection versus Neisseria gonorrhoeae infection among women with pelvic inflammatory disease. Clin Infect Dis 2009;48(1):41–7.
12. Chan PA, Robinette A, Montgomery M, et al. Extragenital Infections Caused by Chlamydia trachomatis and Neisseria gonorrhoeae: A Review of the Literature. Infect Dis Obstet Gynecol 2016;2016:5758387.
13. Pathan E, Inman RD. Pathophysiology of Reactive Arthritis. In: Espinoza LR, editor. Infections and the rheumatic diseases. Cham: Springer International Publishing; 2019. p. 345–53.

14. Vallely LM, Egli-Gany D, Wand H, et al. Adverse pregnancy and neonatal outcomes associated with Neisseria gonorrhoeae: systematic review and meta-analysis. Sex Transm Infect 2021;97(2):104–11.

15. Adachi KN, Nielsen-Saines K, Klausner JD. Chlamydia trachomatis Screening and Treatment in Pregnancy to Reduce Adverse Pregnancy and Neonatal Outcomes: A Review. Front Public Health 2021;9:531073.

16. Ryan GM Jr, Abdella TN, McNeeley SG, et al. Chlamydia trachomatis infection in pregnancy and effect of treatment on outcome. Am J Obstet Gynecol 1990; 162(1):34–9.

17. Baud D, Goy G, Jaton K, et al. Role of Chlamydia trachomatis in miscarriage. Emerg Infect Dis 2011;17(9):1630–5.

18. Burdette ER, Young MR, Dude CM, et al. Association of Delayed Treatment of Chlamydial Infection and Gonorrhea in Pregnancy and Preterm Birth. Sex Transm Dis 2021;48(12):925–31.

19. Hoffman BL, Schorge JO, Halvorson LM, et al. Gynecologic infection. Williams Gynecology. 4edition. New York, NY: McGraw-Hill Education; 2020.

20. USPST Force, Davidson KW, Barry MJ, et al. Screening for Chlamydia and Gonorrhea: US Preventive Services Task Force Recommendation Statement. JAMA 2021;326(10):949–56.

21. Jann JT, Cunningham NJ, Assaf RD, et al. Evidence supporting the standardisation of extragenital gonorrhoea and chlamydia screenings for women. Sex Transm Infect 2021;97(8):601–6.

22. Dang CM, Pao J, Taherzadeh D, et al. Paired Testing of Sexually Transmitted Infections With Urine Pregnancy Tests in Incarcerated Women. Sex Transm Dis 2021;48(8S):S20–5.

23. Oakeshott P, Kerry S, Aghaizu A, et al. Randomised controlled trial of screening for Chlamydia trachomatis to prevent pelvic inflammatory disease: the POPI (prevention of pelvic infection) trial. BMJ 2010;340:c1642.

24. Scholes D, Stergachis A, Heidrich FE, et al. Prevention of pelvic inflammatory disease by screening for cervical chlamydial infection. N Engl J Med 1996;334(21): 1362–6.

25. Hocking JS, Temple-Smith M, Guy R, et al. Population effectiveness of opportunistic chlamydia testing in primary care in Australia: a cluster-randomised controlled trial. Lancet 2018;392(10156):1413–22.

26. Knox J, Tabrizi SN, Miller P, et al. Evaluation of self-collected samples in contrast to practitioner-collected samples for detection of Chlamydia trachomatis, Neisseria gonorrhoeae, and Trichomonas vaginalis by polymerase chain reaction among women living in remote areas. Sex Transm Dis 2002;29(11):647–54.

27. Masek BJ, Arora N, Quinn N, et al. Performance of three nucleic acid amplification tests for detection of Chlamydia trachomatis and Neisseria gonorrhoeae by use of self-collected vaginal swabs obtained via an Internet-based screening program. J Clin Microbiol 2009;47(6):1663–7.

28. Division of STD Prevention NCfH. Viral Hepatitis, STD, and TB Prevention. Gonococcal Infections Among Adolescents and Adults. Secondary gonococcal infections among adolescents and adults. 2021. Available at: https://www.cdc.gov/std/treatment-guidelines/gonorrhea-adults.htm.

29. Division of STD Prevention NCfH. Viral Hepatitis, STD, and TB Prevention. Chlamydia Infections. Secondary Chlamydia Infections. 2021. Available at: https://www.cdc.gov/std/treatment-guidelines/chlamydia.htm.

30. Kong FY, Tabrizi SN, Law M, et al. Azithromycin versus doxycycline for the treatment of genital chlamydia infection: a meta-analysis of randomized controlled trials. Clin Infect Dis 2014;59(2):193–205.

31. Dukers-Muijrers N, Wolffs PFG, De Vries H, et al. Treatment Effectiveness of Azithromycin and Doxycycline in Uncomplicated Rectal and Vaginal Chlamydia trachomatis Infections in Women: A Multicenter Observational Study (FemCure). Clin Infect Dis 2019;69(11):1946–54.

32. Dombrowski JC, Wierzbicki MR, Newman LM, et al. Doxycycline Versus Azithromycin for the Treatment of Rectal Chlamydia in Men Who Have Sex With Men: A Randomized Controlled Trial. Clin Infect Dis 2021;73(5):824–31.

33. Barbee LA, St Cyr SB. Management of Neisseria gonorrhoeae in the United States: Summary of Evidence From the Development of the 2020 Gonorrhea Treatment Recommendations and the 2021 Centers for Disease Control and Prevention Sexually Transmitted Infection Treatment Guidelines. Clin Infect Dis 2022; 74(Suppl_2):S95–111.

34. St Cyr S, Barbee L, Workowski KA, et al. Update to CDC's Treatment Guidelines for Gonococcal Infection, 2020. MMWR Morb Mortal Wkly Rep 2020;69(50): 1911–6.

35. Division of STD. Prevention NCfH; Viral Hepatitis, STD, and TB Prevention, Sexually transmitted disease surveillance 2019: gonococcal isolate survellience Project (GISP) supplement and profiles. Atlanta, Georgia: Department of Health and Human Services; 2021.

36. ACOG Committee Opinion No. 737: expedited partner therapy. Obstet Gynecol 2018;131(6):e190–3.

37. Division of STD Prevention NCfH. Viral Hepatitis, STD, and TB prevention. legal status of expedited partner therapy. secondary legal status of expedited partner therapy. 2021. Available at: https://www.cdc.gov/std/ept/legal/default.htm#a3.

38. Golden MR, Whittington WL, Handsfield HH, et al. Effect of expedited treatment of sex partners on recurrent or persistent gonorrhea or chlamydial infection. N Engl J Med 2005;352(7):676–85.

39. Jamison CD, Coleman JS, Mmeje O. Improving women's health and combatting sexually transmitted infections through expedited partner therapy. Obstet Gynecol 2019;133(3):416–22.

40. Nelson T, Nandwani J, Johnson D. Gonorrhea and chlamydia cases are rising in the united states: expedited partner therapy might help. Sex Transm Dis 2022; 49(1):e1–3.

41. Jamison CD, Waselewski M, Gogineni V, et al. Youth knowledge and perspectives on expedited partner therapy. J Adolesc Health 2022;70(1):114–9.

42. Vaidya S, Johnson K, Rogers M, et al. Predictors of index patient acceptance of expedited partner therapy for Chlamydia trachomatis infection and reasons for refusal, sexually transmitted disease clinics, New York City, 2011 to 2012. Sex Transm Dis 2014;41(11):690–4.

43. Oglesby A, Ricke I, Swenson A, et al. Women's knowledge and hypothetical acceptance of expedited partner therapy for chlamydia. Sex Health 2022; 18(6):502–7.

44. Okah E, Westheimer EF, Jamison K, et al. Frequency of nucleic acid amplification test positivity among men who have sex with men returning for a test-of-cure visit 7 to 30 days after treatment of laboratory-confirmed neisseria gonorrhoeae infection at 2 public sexual health clinics, New York City, 2013 to 2016. Sex Transm Dis 20 18;45(3):177–82.

45. Barbee LA, Golden MR. Editorial commentary: when to perform a test of cure for gonorrhea: controversies and evolving data. Clin Infect Dis 2016;62(11):1356–9.
46. Radcliffe KW, Rowen D, Mercey DE, et al. Is a test of cure necessary following treatment for cervical infection with Chlamydia trachomatis? Genitourin Med 1990;66(6):444–6.
47. Jenks JD, Hester L, Ryan E, et al. Test-of-Cure After Treatment of Pharyngeal Gonorrhea in Durham, North Carolina, 2021-2022. Sex Transm Dis 2022;49(10): 677–81.
48. Barbee LA, Soge OO, Khosropour CM, et al. Time to Clearance of Neisseria gonorrhoeae RNA at the Pharynx following Treatment. J Clin Microbiol 2022;60(6): e0039922.
49. Van Der Pol B, Chernesky M, Gaydos CA, et al. Multicenter Comparison of Nucleic Acid Amplification Tests for the Diagnosis of Rectal and Oropharyngeal Chlamydia trachomatis and Neisseria gonorrhoeae Infections. J Clin Microbiol 2022;60(1):e0136321.
50. Bachmann LH, Johnson RE, Cheng H, et al. Nucleic acid amplification tests for diagnosis of Neisseria gonorrhoeae oropharyngeal infections. J Clin Microbiol 2009;47(4):902–7.
51. Lazenby GB, Korte JE, Tillman S, et al. A recommendation for timing of repeat Chlamydia trachomatis test following infection and treatment in pregnant and nonpregnant women. Int J STD AIDS 2017;28(9):902–9.
52. Doxycycline post-exposure prophylaxis for STI prevention among MSM and transgender women on HIV PrEP or living with HIV: high efficacy to reduce incident STI's in a randomized trial. Montreal, Canada: International AIDS Conference; 2022; 2022.
53. Division of STD Prevention NCfH. Viral Hepatitis, STD, and TB Prevention. CDC Response to Doxy-PEP data presented at 2022 International AIDS Conference. Secondary CDC Response to Doxy-PEP data presented at 2022 International AIDS Conference. 2022. Available at: https://www.cdc.gov/nchhstp/newsroom/2022/Doxy-PEP-clinical-data-presented-at-2022-AIDS-Conference.html.

Microbiome and Vulvovaginitis

Anna Maya Powell, MD, MSc[a], Isabella Sarria, BA[b], Oluwatosin Goje, MD, MSCR[c,*]

KEYWORDS

- Bacterial vaginosis • Yeast infection • Trichomoniasis
- Desquamative inflammatory vaginitis • Microbiome • Vaginal dysbiosis

KEY POINTS

- Vulvovaginitis is one of the main reasons reproductive aged women call or visit a provider.
- The authors advocate a multifaceted approach to management of vulvovaginitis using the triad of pharmacologic therapy, lifestyle modification, and education.
- Patients with recurrent bacterial vaginosis and recurrent vulvovaginal candidiasis may benefit from suppressive therapy.
- Trichomoniasis is underreported and is asymptomatic in most of the patients.
- In the menopausal or perimenopausal patient with recurrent vaginal symptoms, consider desquamative inflammatory vaginitis and genitourinary symptom of menopause if antimicrobials are ineffective.

INTRODUCTION

Vulvovaginitis (itching, discharge, and odor) is one of the top reasons patients with vaginas will present to a Gynecologist's office. Most commonly attributed to yeast, bacterial vaginosis, or trichomoniasis, vaginitis is a global health concern that costs patients and the health care system an estimated $4.8 billion annually.[1] Despite patient anecdotes to the contrary, vaginitis symptoms are notoriously nonspecific and do not lend themselves to easy self-diagnosis.[2] Only one-third of women who self-diagnosed vulvovaginal candidiasis (VVC) actually had it, in one study.[2] Getting to the gynecology office can be a critical step in breaking the cycle of bothersome symptoms that affect 15% to 39% of female patients in the United States. This review discusses updates in literature concerning diagnosis and treatment of acute and recurrent vaginitis as well as similar "look-alike" conditions of desquamative inflammatory vaginitis (DIV) and genitourinary syndrome of menopause/atrophic vaginitis

[a] Johns Hopkins University School of Medicine, 600 North Wolfe Street, Phipps 249, Baltimore, MD 21287, USA; [b] Johns Hopkins University Bloomberg School of Public Health, 615 North Wolfe Street, Baltimore, MD 21205, USA; [c] OB/GYN and Women's Health Institute, Cleveland Clinic Foundation, 9500 Euclid Avenue, A81, Cleveland, OH 44195, USA
* Corresponding author.
E-mail address: gojeo@ccf.org
Twitter: @annapbanana (A.M.P.); @goje_dr (O.G.)

Obstet Gynecol Clin N Am 50 (2023) 311–326
https://doi.org/10.1016/j.ogc.2023.02.005
0889-8545/23/© 2023 Elsevier Inc. All rights reserved.
obgyn.theclinics.com

through the lens of the vaginal microbiome and offer expert guidance to make management less daunting. It is important to note that not all patients presenting with vaginitis symptoms will identify as women. Trans men, nonbinary, and intersex individuals may also experience vaginitis. If cis-women language is used, this reflects what is reported in the literature and is not intended as erasure of this demographic.

INFECTIOUS CAUSE
Bacterial Vaginosis

Bacterial vaginosis (BV) is the most common cause of vaginitis worldwide. BV has been linked to preterm delivery, increase in intraamniotic infection, endometritis, post-abortal infection, and vaginal cuff cellulitis following a hysterectomy.[3] BV has also been associated with increased risk factor for human immunodeficiency virus (HIV) infection.[4] BV is associated with vaginal dysbiosis resulting from displacement of lactic acid–producing Lactobacillus spp with higher concentrations of facultative and strict anaerobic bacteria including Gardnerella vaginalis, Prevotella spp, Atopobium vaginae, Sneathia spp, and BV-associated bacteria (BVAB).[5] The exact cause of BV remains elusive but newer vaginal microbiome studies attempt to shed light on the vaginal environment that may foster dysbiosis. Although G vaginalis and P bivia are highly abundant in women diagnosed with BV, they induce a less robust inflammatory response from vaginal epithelial cells than secondary colonizers (A vaginae, Sneathia, and other BVAB) that more potently stimulate host immunity.[6,7] BV is thought to be associated with biofilm formation, which in particular makes recurrent disease so difficult to treat.[7–9] Biofilms are surface-attached cells of microbes encased in a self-produced extracellular matrix.[10] Studies have shown that metronidazole may temporarily break up biofilm, which quickly regenerates itself with therapy completion, demonstrating a large reservoir of bacteria that persist following treatment cessation.[11] Biofilms are implicated in both BV and VVC, particularly in the setting of treatment failure and symptomatic recurrence.[10]

Role of the microbiome in bacterial vaginosis

The vagina of healthy persons is host to microbial colonization, with Lactobacillus playing a major role (95%).[12] Based on the different species of specific Lactobacillus, it can be divided into 5 different community state types (CSTs).[13] Among them, CST I, II, III, and V are mainly Lactobacillus crispatus, Lactobacillus gasseri, Lactobacillus Iners, and Lactobacillus Jensenii, respectively, whereas CST IV is anaerobe dominant.[14,15] L crispatus, L gasseri, and L jensenii produce lactic acid and H_2O_2, acidify the vaginal environment to pH less than 4.5, and inhibit the growth of other viruses and bacteria.[16,17] In addition, the metabolites produced by Lactobacillus can also stimulate the host to produce antimicrobial peptides and antiinflammatory cytokines.[18] Vaginal epithelial cells change periodically under the action of estrogen and progesterone. Glycogen produced in this process provides energy for the growth of Lactobacillus. Furthermore, recurrence rate of BV after oral metronidazole treatment is very high, and the systemic use of antibiotics has great side effects.[6,19]

Diagnosis

BV presents classically with a watery gray homogenous discharge, often accompanied by a "fishy" amine odor. Initial evaluation in the office should include pH test and microscopy, if available. The use of Amsel's criteria or gram stain with Nugent score (limited to research setting) is recommended,[20,21] with Amsel facilitating a clinical diagnosis and treatment initiation in the office (**Table 1**). Routine bacterial culture of the vagina is not recommended because normal vaginal flora is heterogeneous.

Table 1
Summary of key points in diagnosis and treatment of vulvovaginitis

Condition	Diagnosis	First-Line Treatment	New Therapy	Notes
Bacterial vaginosis	Amsel criteria[a] Molecular testing	Oral or vaginal nitroimidazole, oral or vaginal clindamycin Lifestyle modification	Lactin-V TOL 463	Limited evidence to support partner therapy
Recurrent BV	≥ 3 documented BV episodes per year	Oral nitroimidazole followed by intravaginal metronidazole OR Oral nitroimidazole followed by intravaginal boric acid and intravaginal metronidazole	—	May consider referral to specialist See **Fig. 1**.
Vulvovaginal candidiasis	Microscopy Molecular testing Fungal culture[a]	Oral or vaginal azole Lifestyle modification	Ibrexafungerp Oteseconazole **Box 1**	—
Recurrent VVC	≥ 3 documented VVC episodes per year	3 doses of oral or vaginal azole followed by weekly fluconazole for up to 6 months Intravaginal boric acid nightly x 21 days followed by twice weekly vaginal administration	Oteseconazole	May consider referral to specialist Consider speciation and resistance testing with fungal culture
Trichomonas vaginalis (TV)	Microscopy Molecular testing[a]	Oral nitroimidazole, eg, Metronidazole, 500 mg, BID x 7 days Expedited partner therapy	n/a	Extended dosing now recommended for women with/without HIV

(continued on next page)

Table 1
(continued)

Condition	Diagnosis	First-Line Treatment	New Therapy	Notes
Recurrent TV	Culture Documented treatment failure after ruling out reinfection	See CDC STI 2021 Guidelines for suggested treatment algorithm See **Box 2**	—	May consider referral to specialist especially in cases of nitroimidazole allergy Refer to CDC guidelines for nitroimidazole resistance testing
Desquamative Inflammatory Vaginitis	Clinical findings plus microscopy	Vaginal hydrocortisone or clindamycin	—	—
Genitourinary syndrome of menopause (GSM)	Clinical findings plus microscopy	estrogen formulation	—	—

[a] Denotes gold-standard method of diagnosis.

- *Point of care*: BV is diagnosed using Amsel's criteria (presence of 3 out of 4 of these criteria: pH > 4.5, positive whiff test with KOH application, homogenous discharge, and presence of ≥20% clue cells).
- *Molecular testing*: Although Amsel's criteria are the preferred method and cost-effective, the Food and Drug Administration (FDA) has approved commercial tests that are readily available in offices.[20]

The AFFIRM VP III (Becton Dickinson), a nonamplified nucleic acid probe hybridization test for detection of *T vaginalis*, *Candida spp*, *and G vaginalis*, is used in the office because of its simplicity of collection and rapid turnover. When AFFIRM VP III was compared with nucleic acid amplification–based assay (BV-polymerase chain reaction [PCR]) in a cohort of 323 symptomatic women, BV-PCR was 96.9% sensitive and 92.6% specific for BV, whereas AFFIRM was 90.1% sensitive and 67.6% specific.[22]

Management

Patients with symptomatic BV should be treated based on the 2021 CDC's Sexually Transmitted Infections (STI) Treatment Guidelines[20]: metronidazole, 500 mg, orally 2 times a day for 7 days, or metronidazole 0.75% (5 g) intravaginal gel daily for 5 days, or clindamycin 2% gel (5 g) intravaginal for 7 days. In this subsection, the authors focus on patients with recurrent BV (RBV) (**Fig. 1**). RBV is defined as 3 or more documented episodes within 1 year. The frequency of symptomatic episodes may be difficult to treat, often leading to patients' frustration.[23] Bacterial vaginosis may recur in up to 30% of patients within 3 months and 58% within 12 months.[24] Goje and colleagues[19] in a pilot project looked at the effect of oral metronidazole on the vaginal microbiome of patients with RBV and demonstrated the beneficial effect of metronidazole was temporary, with recurrence by day 30 after metronidazole therapy. Drivers of recurrence and behaviors that increase the risk of RBV should be discussed with patient, such as avoidance of vaginal douching and correct and consistent condom use during intercourse. In addition, challenges and opportunities to prevent recurrence in sexually active persons should be discussed.[24,25] Sobel and colleagues describe use of metronidazole vaginal gel for RBV suppression in a multicenter prospective trial. During suppressive therapy, the relative risk of RBV for participants on suppressive therapy was 0.43 (by MITT analysis, CI = 0.25–0.73), with probability for continued cure of 70% for metronidazole arm (declining to 34%, compared with 39% and 18%, respectively) by 28 weeks follow-up.[20] Reichman and colleagues[26] report use

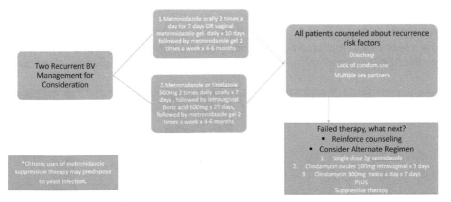

Fig. 1. Clinician's approach to management of recurrent BV. (*Data from* Sobel JD, Ferris D, Schwebke J, et al. Suppressive antibacterial therapy with 0.75% metronidazole vaginal gel to prevent recurrent bacterial vaginosis. Am J Obstet Gynecol. May 2006;194(5):1283-9. https://doi.org/10.1016/j.ajog.2005.11.041.)

of nitroimidazole for 7 to 10 days followed by intravaginal boric acid (IBA) supposi- tories daily for 21 days and subsequent vaginal metronidazole suppression therapy twice weekly for 16 weeks.[27] In this study, cure after nitroimidazole therapy and IBA ranged from 88% to 92%, 7 and 12 weeks after the initial visit. Cumulative cure rates at 12, 16, and 28 weeks from initial visit were 87%, 78%, and 65% with a failure rate of 50% by 36 weeks follow-up.

Newer therapeutics and considerations

Research is ongoing for nonantibiotic therapy. A randomized, double-blind, placebo- controlled phase 2b trial sought to evaluate efficacy of L crispatus CTV-05 (Lactin-V) in preventing recurrent bacterial vaginosis.[28] The primary outcome of the study was per- centage of women with BV recurrence by week 12 with follow-up study investigating up to 24 weeks after treatment.[28] Use of Lactin-V after vaginal metronidazole treat- ment resulted in significantly lower incidence of RBV compared to placebo at 12 weeks (ITT risk ratio 0.66, 95% CI 0.44–0.87.). Lactin-V was also associated with significantly lower concentrations of proinflammatory cytokine interleukin-1α and soluble E-cad- herin, a marker of epithelial barrier disruption.[29] TOL-463 (Boric acid, EDTA), another medication in development, was tested in a phase 2 randomized, investigator-blinded trial conducted at 2 sexual health clinics to evaluate women with BV or VVC. TOL-463 was effective and safe in treating BV and VVC, and its role as a biofilm disrupter should be explored. IBA in general has become widely available as an over-the-counter medi- cation. The limited safety data are overall reassuring for use in nonpregnant women of reproductive age,[30] although it is recommended that patients review IBA use with a clinician before starting therapy and avoid pregnancy while using this treatment.

Vulvovaginal Candidiasis

Vulvo-vaginal candidiasis (VVC) is the second most common cause of vulvovaginitis and clinically diagnosed based on the presence of vaginal discharge, external dysuria, vulvar pruritis, pain, swelling, or redness. Signs include vulvar edema, fissures, exco- riations, and sometimes thick curdy vaginal discharge (**Fig. 2**A&B); 75% of women are affected at least once in their lifetime, and more than 130 million women are affected by VVC annually worldwide.[31] An online survey conducted in the United States and 5 European countries reported that 20% had experienced at least one episode of VVC, 45% had 2 to 5 recurrences, and 29% had 5 to 20 episodes in their lifetime.[27,32] Although various risk factors for VVC have been outlined, greater than 50% have no risk factors identified.[12,21,25]

Role of the microbiome

The role of vaginal microbiome (VMB) composition in VVC is unclear and needs further studies. Only a small number of vaginal bacteria were strongly and significantly

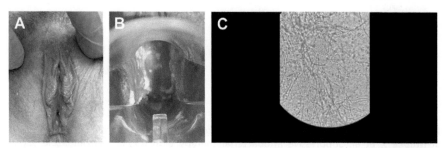

Fig. 2. (A) Vulvar yeast infection. (B) Yeast vaginitis. (C) Fungal elements on microscopy.

associated with the presence or absence of yeast.[33] Literature has reported normal vaginal pH (pH ~ 4.5) during VVC, indicating the presence of sufficient number of *Lactobacilli* to maintain the acidification of vagina.[23] Additional studies found that *Lactobacillus* dominance seems to be maintained with no difference in VMB composition in women with and without VVC.[28,34,35] These findings suggest that the presence of *Lactobacilli* in women with VVC do not play a critical role in defending against VVC.[28]

Diagnosis
Candida albicans accounts for 85% to -95% of VVC.[36–39] Saline microscopy with the addition of 10% KOH is 50% sensitivity when available and fungal culture remains the gold standard for diagnosis[40,41] (see **Table1**).

- *Point of care*: *saline microscopy with KOH*, if available, offers the ability to make a diagnosis in the office and start treatment immediately.[41] Office diagnosis includes symptoms, ± signs, and positive wet prep demonstrating budding yeasts, hyphae, or pseudohyphae (**Fig. 2**C).
- *Gold standard*: *fungal culture*: patients with recurrent or complicated VVC (**Table 2**) or suspected antifungal resistance/treatment failure should be offered a fungal culture. The culprit could be *non-albicans Candida* such as *Candida Glabrata* that may not be sensitive to the azoles or fluconazole resistance.[21,27,39,42,43] Patients with negative wet prep but existing signs or symptoms should be offered a culture and empiric treatment considered if symptomatic.
- *Molecular testing*: the Affirm VP-III (Becton Dickinson) can produce comparable results to traditionally collected sample. The CAN-PCR is a multiplexed, real-time, PCR assay, and its performance was compared with the Affirm VPIII in diagnosis of candida by Cartwright and colleagues.[22] Affirm *Candida* spp assay had a sensitivity of 58.1% and specificity of 100%, whereas the CAN-PCR assay resulted in a sensitivity of 97.7% and specificity of 93.2% in a cohort of 102 patients using 43 patients with a positive yeast culture as the referent group.

Management
We advocate a multifaceted approach to management of VVC using the triad of pharmacologic therapy, lifestyle modification, and education in order to optimize risk factor reduction (eg, glycemic control in diabetes). According to the 2021 CDC guidelines, oral or vaginal azoles remain the most commonly prescribed therapeutics for VVC and provide effective relief in most of the patients.[20]

- *Recurrent/Resistance*: recurrent VVC (RVVC) can be problematic and carry social and psychological consequences for affected patients. RVVC is defined as 3 or

Table 2
Classification of vulvovaginal candidiasis

Uncomplicated	Complicated
Sporadic or infrequent infections (<3 in 12 mo)	Recurrent episode (≥3 in 12 mo)
Mild to moderate symptoms or findings	Severe symptoms or findings
Candida albicans infection	*Non-albicans Candida*
Nonimmunocompromised patient	Diabetes mellitus, immunosuppressive condition or therapy

Data from Sobel JD, Faro S, Force RW, et al. Vulvovaginal candidiasis: epidemiologic, diagnostic, and therapeutic considerations. Am J Obstet Gynecol. Feb 1998;178(2):203-11. https://doi.org/10.1016/s0002-9378(98)80001 x.

more episodes of symptomatic VVC in 1 year. Although the pathogenesis of RVVC is poorly understood,[12,21,25] increasing azole resistance has been reported in *C albicans* isolates.[44] Prolonged course of the topical azoles for 7 to 14 days or oral fluconazole 150 mg every 3 days for a total of 3 doses has been successful in RVVC. Prolonged course of a nonfluconazole azole or intravaginal Boric acid, 600 mg, daily for 3 weeks maybe effective. Patients with RVVC should be offered oral fluconazole, 150 mg, weekly for 6 months as maintenance regimen after the initial therapy.[45] If not feasible, intermittent topical therapy should be considered. In addition to the azoles, newer medications are available for this cohort.[23] Ibrexafungerp is the first triterpenoid class antifungal and has a similar mechanism of action to echinocandins. Schwebke and colleagues report on ibrexafungerp versus placebo in a phase 3, randomized, and controlled superiority trial (VANISH 303). Study participants receiving ibrexafungerp had more frequent clinical cures (50.5% vs 28.6%; P = .001), mycological cure (49.5% vs 19.4%; P < .001), and overall success (30.6% vs 12.6%, P < .001) compared with placebo.[46] Oteseconazole is effective in preventing acute VVC recurrence and treating RVVC. Oral oteseconazole reduced the rate of vaginal yeast recolonization and decreased posttherapy recurrence rates of symptomatic vaginitis.[47] In addition to newer therapeutics, compounded medications including amphotericin B, intravaginal boric acid, and flucytosine have been reported to be effective in non-*albicans candida* vaginitis and recalcitrant and resistant cases[48–51] (**Box 1**).

Trichomoniasis

Trichomonas vaginalis (TV), a flagellated parasitic protozoan, is the most prevalent nonviral STI worldwide and an important vaginitis leading to reproductive morbidity, including HIV acquisition and transmission. Although not reportable, trichomoniasis is more prevalent in Black persons, with highest rates among Black women.[52,53]

Role of the microbiome
Compared with vaginal swabs from patients without trichomoniasis, the vaginal microbiome of samples with TV showed enrichment of various anaerobes including *Megasphera 2*, *Parvimonas*, *Prevotella*, and *Sneathia*.[53,54] Further cluster analysis of

---

Box 1
Alternative regimen for recurrent vulvovaginal candidiasis

Second-line agents and compounded formulations
  Boric acid, 600 mg, intravaginal daily × 21 days
  Flucytosine 15.5% intravaginal (5 g) daily × 14 days
  Amphotericin B vaginal suppositories 50 mg daily × 14 days
  Newer medications that can be used as second-line ibrexafungerp (Brexafemme) 300 mg BID × 1 day
  [a]Oteseconazole (Vivjoa)
  Oteseconazole alone: on day 1: administer VIVJOA, 600 mg (as a single dose), then on day 2: administer VIVJOA 450 mg (as a single dose), then beginning on day 14: administer VIVJOA, 150 mg, once a week (every 7 days) for 11 weeks (weeks 2 through 12).
  Oteseconazole with fluconazole: on day 1, day 4, and day 7: administer fluconazole, 150 mg, orally, then on days 14 through 20: administer VIVJOA, 150 mg, once daily for 7 days, then beginning on day 28: administer VIVJOA, 150 mg, once a week (every 7 days) for 11 weeks (weeks 4 through 14).

Recommend an ID/Vaginitis specialist consultation.[a] Based on manufacturers' prescribing information.

samples with TV revealed 2 unique groups by *Mycoplasma hominis* abundance; those with higher *M hominis* abundance had clinical evidence of vaginal inflammation.[53] Studies show a strong association between TV and BV and both frequently occur as coinfections among women.[14,55] VMB community state types with higher anaerobe dominance (CST-IV) associated with an 8-fold increased odds of detecting *T vaginalis* compared with women in the *L crispatus*-dominated state (odd ratio [OR]:8.26, 95% confidence interval [CI]:1.07–372.65.)[55]

Diagnosis

Most of the patients are asymptomatic, and among those who become symptomatic, symptoms include abnormal vaginal discharge, dysuria, itching, vulvovaginal irritation, and pelvic pain.[23] pH could be variable and on examination patients may have the classic strawberry cervix, erythematous vagina and vestibule, malodorous frothy, or yellow or green discharge. Inflammation is an important feature of TV (**Fig. 3**).

- *Point of care*: *saline microscopy* of motile trichomonads with their characteristic jerky movements is 100% specific and 50% sensitive.[56]
- *Molecular testing*: nucleic acid probe techniques are the most sensitive test and gold standard (see **Table 1**). Aptima Trichomonas vaginalis Assay (Hologic Gen-Probe, San Diego, CA, USA) is cleared for use with urine, endocervical, and vaginal swabs. It has a sensitivity of 95.3% to 100% and specificity 95.2% to 100%[57] compared with microscopy and culture. Multiple FDA-approved rapid tests are also available with improved sensitivities and specificities compared with microscopy; a commonly performed one is the Affirm VP III (Becton, Dickinson & Co.; Franklin Lakes, NJ, USA).[58]

Management

Nitroimidazoles are the only class of medications with clinically demonstrated efficacy against *T vaginalis* infection.[23] Metronidazole, 500 mg, twice a day orally for 7 days is the recommended regimen in women. Tinidazole, 2 g, orally in a single dose is an alternative. Patients should abstain from sex until they and sex partner are treated and should be offered STI screening including HIV test. Retesting is recommended for

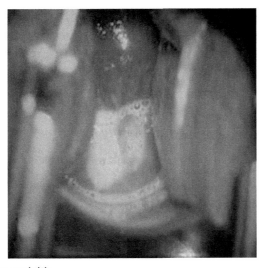

Fig. 3. Trichomonas vaginitis.

all sexually active women lees than 3 months after initial treatment or within 12 months postinitial treatment if the 3 months retesting was not performed.

- *Recurrent/Resistance*: recurrent Trichomoniasis could be from treatment failure, lack of adherence, or reinfection. Reinfection is more common than nitroimidazole resistance. It may occur in the setting of an untreated/infected baseline partner, infection from a new partner, and antibiotic resistance.[59] According to the CDC, data indicate that expedited partner therapy might have a role in partner management for trichomoniasis.[23] If reinfection is suspected, repeat therapy with metronidazole, 500 mg, orally twice a day for 7 days. If patient has no reexposure, consider metronidazole or tinidazole, 2 g, daily for 7 days. Other regimens of high-dose tinidazole oral and vaginal should be discussed with a specialist. For patients with imidazole allergy, desensitization can be performed if appropriate, and if TV remains persistent or patient is allergic to imidazole, patient should be referred to a specialist where intravaginal compounded 4 g of (6.25%) paromomycin may be considered[23] (**Box 2**).

NONINFECTIOUS VAGINITIS

Noninfectious vaginitis could mimic infectious vaginitis and may lead to delay in diagnosis if not considered as a differential. Two of them are discussed briefly in this article.

- *DIV*: it is a chronic vaginal disorder of unknown cause although various microorganisms have been implicated. It is a diagnosis of exclusion. Diagnosis is usually clinical and microscopic. The use of vaginal molecular testing without microscopy may delay diagnosis and subsequently delay appropriate therapy. Menopausal women who are not sexually active and persistently complain of vaginal signs and symptoms despite multiple antimicrobial therapy should have microscopy performed or referred to a specialist. The average patient is a perimenopausal or menopausal woman complaining of recurrent or persistent copious mucoid, green-yellow discharge.[60,61] Other associated features include vulvar and vaginal pain, itching, redness, vaginal spotting, postcoital spotting, and dyspareunia. On examination the vulva may be erythematous, friable, and tender to touch. The vagina may be diffusely erythematous (**Fig. 4**A). The vaginal pH is greater than 4.5. Saline microscopy shows leukorrhea and sometimes increased parabasal cells (**Fig. 4**B).

Box 2
Treatment of recurrent trichomoniasis

Rule out resistance via a CDC consult
  Tinidazole oral 2–3 g daily × 10–14 days
  Tinidazole oral 500 mg daily × 4 days PLUS Tinidazole vaginal 500 mg twice a day for 14 days
  Paromomycin 15% (5 g) bedtime × 14 days
  Tinidazole 1 g × 3 days plus 5 g of 15% paromomycin cream nightly × 14 days

Patient should be referred to a vaginitis or infectious disease specialist for high-dose imidazole or compounded paromomycin management.

Data from Workowski KA, Bachmann LH, Chan PA, et al. Sexually Transmitted Infections Treatment Guidelines, 2021. MMWR Recomm Rep. Jul 23 2021;70(4):1-187. https://doi.org/10.15585/mmwr.rr7004a1.

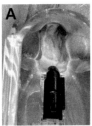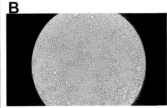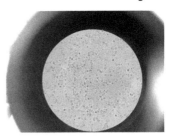

Fig. 4. (*A*) Desquamative inflammatory vaginitis (creamy vaginal discharge with erythema of vagina). (*B*) Desquamative inflammatory vaginitis (microscopy with leukorrhea and parabasal cells).

Diagnosis

- At least 1 symptom (abnormal vaginal discharge, dyspareunia, pruritus, pain, irritation, or burning) AND
- Vaginal inflammation on examination AND
- pH greater than 4.5 AND
- Presence of leukorrhea ± parabsasal cells

Management

There is a deficit of research for DIV; however, the first-line therapy is intravaginal 2% clindamycin daily for 4 to 6 weeks and second-line 10% intravaginal hydrocortisone (hydrocortisone maybe compounded with 2% clindamycin and estrogen cream if vagina is hypoestrogenic).[60,61] Patient should be counseled about risk of treatment failure and need for prolonged treatment. Patients should be managed by a specialist or provider with knowledge on DIV.

- *Genitourinary syndrome of menopause (GSM)*: often seen in menopausal or hypoestrogenic women (breastfeeding, medical or surgical menopause). Postmenopausal women with recurrent vaginal complaints despite antimicrobial or antifungal therapy should be evaluated for GSM. Clinical feature may include persistent vulvovaginal itching, serous discharge, pain, burning, and dyspareunia.[62] Patients may have a secondary fungal or bacterial infection and present with a history of temporary relief during or after therapy with recurrence of symptoms posttreatment.
- *Microbiome*: the VMB of menopausal women reflects a low estrogen environment and is more anaerobe dominant.[52] *Lactobacillus spp* decline during menopause and may affect the extent of GSM in patients. One study identified that postmenopausal women with *L gasseri–/L jensenii*–dominant communities had the lowest odds of vaginal dryness (OR 0.36; 95%CI 0.12–1.06) and low libido (OR 0.28, 95%CI 0.10–0.74) compared with women with more anaerobic dominance.[53]
- *Diagnosis*: examination may reveal atrophic vulvar and vaginal mucosa. Vaginal mucosa may seem pale, lacking rugae or elasticity.
- Saline microscopy may reveal paucity of vaginal epithelial cells, white blood cells, and parabasal cells. Vaginal pH is usually greater than 4.5.
- *Management*: infection should be considered and treated as needed and vaginal or systemic hormonal therapy recommended based on *NAMS* guidance.[62]

ROLE OF PROBIOTICS

Historically, there has been mixed data supporting use of probiotics as a treatment or adjuvant for vaginitis, as treatment effects in the vagina are limited and do not seem to recolonize the vagina with favorable microbiota.[63] Factors that may affect the overall success of probiotics include the formulation of *Lactobacillus*, route of administration, intercourse during treatment, ability of the supplemental bacteria to colonize vaginal epithelium, and the patient's resident microbiota.[64] Overall, newer probiotics formulated with proven lactobacillus formulations may prove a beneficial addition to the treatment armament for vaginitis. The role of probiotics in prevention or management of infectious vaginitis requires further research.

CLINICS CARE POINTS

- BV-PCR testing of Gardnerella amplification is insufficient to accurately diagnose BV and is no longer recommended.
- Published regimens for management of RBV use a nitroimidazole induction course followed by maintenance therapy with either vaginal metronidazole or boric acid for up to 6 months. Recurrence rates during maintenance therapy are typically low, whereas the rates increase with treatment cessation.
- Fungal culture can be used to diagnose azole-resistant *Candida albicans* isolates or non-*albicans Candida* isolates for patients with difficult-to-treat yeast vaginitis.
- Reinfection is the most common reason for positive Trichomonas test of cure; ensuring partners are treated appropriately and intercourse is avoided until treatment completion is key.
- DIV requires clinical diagnosis *supported* by microscopy. Prolonged treatment with clindamycin or hydrocortisone may be necessary to resolve symptoms.
- Genitourinary syndrome of menopause is very common in postmenopausal women. Microscopic findings of parabasal cells can help *support* this diagnosis. Vaginal estrogen formulations are considered best treatment.

DISCLOSURE

Dr O. Goje receives honorarium from Merck Manual Professionals, Up-To-Date, Elsevier Clinical Key, and Scynexis. Dr A.M. Powell and Ms I. Sarria have nothing to disclose.

REFERENCES

1. Peebles K, Velloza J, Balkus JE, et al. High global burden and costs of bacterial vaginosis: a systematic review and meta-analysis. Sex Transm Dis 2019;46(5): 304–11.
2. Ferris DG, Nyirjesy P, Sobel JD, et al. Over-the-counter antifungal drug misuse associated with patient-diagnosed vulvovaginal candidiasis. Obstet Gynecol 2002;99(3):419–25.
3. Murphy K, Mitchell CM. The interplay of host immunity, environment and the risk of bacterial vaginosis and associated reproductive health outcomes. J Infect Dis 2016;214(Suppl 1):S29–35.
4. Atashili J, Poole C, Ndumbe PM, et al. Bacterial vaginosis and HIV acquisition: a meta-analysis of published studies. AIDS 2008;22:1493–501.
5. Morrill S, Gilbert NM, Lewis AL. Gardnerella vaginalis as a cause of bacterial vaginosis: appraisal of the evidence from in vivo models. Front Cell Infect Microbiol 2020;10:168.

6. Muzny CA, Łaniewski P, Schwebke JR, et al. Host-vaginal microbiota interactions in the pathogenesis of bacterial vaginosis. Curr Opin Infect Dis 2020; 33(1):59–65.

7. Verstraelen H, Swidsinski A. The biofilm in bacterial vaginosis: implications for epidemiology, diagnosis and treatment: 2018 update. Curr Opin Infect Dis 2019;32(1):38–42.

8. Amabebe E, Anumba DOC. Mechanistic insights into immune suppression and evasion in bacterial vaginosis. Curr Microbiol 2022;79(3):84.

9. Swidsinski A, Loening-Baucke V, Mendling W, et al. Infection through structured polymicrobial Gardnerella biofilms (StPM-GB). Histol Histopathol 2014;29(5): 567–87.

10. Muzny CA, Schwebke JR. Biofilms: an underappreciated mechanism of treatment failure and recurrence in vaginal infections. Clin Infect Dis 2015;61(4): 601–6.

11. Swidsinski A, Mendling W, Loening-Baucke V, et al. An adherent Gardnerella vaginalis biofilm persists on the vaginal epithelium after standard therapy with oral metronidazole. Am J Obstet Gynecol 2008;198(1):97.e1–6.

12. Sobel JD. Vulvovaginal candidosis. Lancet 2007;369(9577):1961–71.

13. Ravel J, Gajer P, Abdo Z, et al. Vaginal microbiome of reproductive-age women. Proc Natl Acad Sci U S A 2011;108(Suppl 1):4680–7.

14. Borgogna JC, Shardell MD, Santori EK, et al. The vaginal metabolome and microbiota of cervical HPV-positive and HPV-negative women: a cross-sectional analysis. Bjog 2020;127(2):182–92.

15. Langner CA, Ortiz AM, Flynn JK, et al. The vaginal microbiome of nonhuman primates can be only transiently altered to become lactobacillus dominant without reducing inflammation. Microbiol Spectr 2021;9(3):e0107421.

16. Anderson DJ, Marathe J, Pudney J. The structure of the human vaginal stratum corneum and its role in immune defense. Am J Reprod Immunol 2014;71(6): 618–23.

17. Das S, Bhattacharjee MJ, Mukherjee AK, et al. Recent advances in understanding of multifaceted changes in the vaginal microenvironment: implications in vaginal health and therapeutics. Crit Rev Microbiol 2022;21:1–27.

18. Niu XX, Li T, Zhang X, et al. Lactobacillus crispatus modulates vaginal epithelial cell innate response to candida albicans. Chin Med J (Engl) 2017;130(3): 273–9.

19. Goje O, Shay EO, Markwei M, et al. The effect of oral metronidazole on the vaginal microbiome of patients with recurrent bacterial vaginosis: a pilot investigational study. Human Microbiome Journal 2021;20:100081.

20. Sobel JD, Ferris D, Schwebke J, et al. Suppressive antibacterial therapy with 0.75% metronidazole vaginal gel to prevent recurrent bacterial vaginosis. Am J Obstet Gynecol 2006;194(5):1283–9.

21. Yano J, Sobel JD, Nyirjesy P, et al. Current patient perspectives of vulvovaginal candidiasis: incidence, symptoms, management and post-treatment outcomes. BMC Wom Health 2019;19(1):48.

22. Cartwright CP, Lembke BD, Ramachandran K, et al. Comparison of nucleic acid amplification assays with BD affirm VPIII for diagnosis of vaginitis in symptomatic women. J Clin Microbiol 2013;51(11):3694–9.

23. Workowski KA, Bachmann LH, Chan PA, et al. Sexually transmitted infections treatment guidelines, 2021. MMWR Recomm Rep (Morb Mortal Wkly Rep) 2021;70(4):1–187.

24. Powell AM, Nyirjesy P. Recurrent vulvovaginitis. Best Pract Res Clin Obstet Gynaecol 2014;28(7):967–76.
25. Nyirjesy P, Zhao Y, Ways K, et al. Evaluation of vulvovaginal symptoms and Candida colonization in women with type 2 diabetes mellitus treated with canagliflozin, a sodium glucose co-transporter 2 inhibitor. Curr Med Res Opin 2012; 28(7):1173–8.
26. Reichman O, Akins R, Sobel JD. Boric acid addition to suppressive antimicrobial therapy for recurrent bacterial vaginosis. Sex Transm Dis 2009;36(11):732 4.
27. Azie N, Angulo D, Dehn B, et al. Oral Ibrexafungerp: an investigational agent for the treatment of vulvovaginal candidiasis. Expert Opin Investig Drugs 2020;29(9): 893–900.
28. Wu W, Liao Q, Liu Z. Analysis of the vaginal microecology in patients with severe vulvovaginal candidiasis. Article. Biomed Res 2017;28(1):118–21.
29. Armstrong E, Hemmerling A, Miller S, et al. Sustained effect of LACTIN-V (Lactobacillus crispatus CTV-05) on genital immunology following standard bacterial vaginosis treatment: results from a randomised, placebo-controlled trial. Lancet Microbe 2022;3(6):e435–42.
30. Mittelstaedt R, Kretz A, Levine M, et al. Data on safety of intravaginal boric acid use in pregnant and nonpregnant women: a narrative review. Sex Transm Dis 2021;48(12):e241–7.
31. Denning DW, Kneale M, Sobel JD, et al. Global burden of recurrent vulvovaginal candidiasis: a systematic review. Lancet Infect Dis 2018;18(11):e339–47.
32. Johnson SR, Griffiths H, Humberstone FJ. Attitudes and experience of women to common vaginal infections. J Low Genit Tract Dis 2010;14(4):287–94.
33. Eastment MC, Balkus JE, Richardson BA, et al. Association between vaginal bacterial microbiota and vaginal yeast colonization. J Infect Dis 2021;223(5):914–23.
34. Zhou X, Westman R, Hickey R, et al. Vaginal microbiota of women with frequent vulvovaginal candidiasis. Infect Immun 2009;77(9):4130–5.
35. Vylkova S, Carman AJ, Danhof HA, et al. The fungal pathogen Candida albicans autoinduces hyphal morphogenesis by raising extracellular pH. mBio 2011;2(3). https://doi.org/10.1128/mBio.00055-11. e00055-11.
36. Sobel JD. Recurrent vulvovaginal candidiasis. Am J Obstet Gynecol 2016;214(1): 15–21.
37. Willems HME, Ahmed SS, Liu J, et al. Vulvovaginal candidiasis: a current understanding and burning questions. J Fungi (Basel) 2020;6(1). https://doi.org/10.3390/jof6010027.
38. Achkar JM, Fries BC. Candida infections of the genitourinary tract. Clin Microbiol Rev 2010;23(2):253–73.
39. Gonçalves B, Ferreira C, Alves CT, et al. Vulvovaginal candidiasis: epidemiology, microbiology and risk factors. Crit Rev Microbiol 2016;42(6):905–27.
40. Eckert LO. Clinical practice. Acute vulvovaginitis. N Engl J Med 2006;355(12): 1244–52.
41. Eckert LO, Hawes SE, Stevens CE, et al. Vulvovaginal candidiasis: clinical manifestations, risk factors, management algorithm. Obstet Gynecol 1998;92(5):757–65.
42. Makanjuola O, Bongomin F, Fayemiwo SA. An Update on the Roles of Non-albicans Candida Species in Vulvovaginitis. J Fungi (Basel) 2018;4(4). https://doi.org/10.3390/jof4040121.
43. Vaginitis in Nonpregnant Patients: ACOG Practice Bulletin, Number 215. Obstet Gynecol 2020;135(1):e1–17.
44. Esfahani A, Omran AN, Salehi Z, et al. Molecular epidemiology, antifungal susceptibility, and ERG11 gene mutation of Candida species isolated from vulvovaginal

candidiasis: comparison between recurrent and non-recurrent infections. Microb Pathog 2022;170:105696.

45. Sobel JD, Wiesenfeld HC, Martens M, et al. Maintenance fluconazole therapy for recurrent vulvovaginal candidiasis. N Engl J Med 2004;351(9):876–83.

46. Schwebke JR, Sobel R, Gersten JK, et al. Ibrexafungerp versus placebo for vulvovaginal candidiasis treatment: a phase 3, randomized, controlled superiority trial (VANISH 303). Clin Infect Dis 2022;74(11):1979–85.

47. Sobel JD, Donders G, Degenhardt T, et al. Efficacy and safety of oteseconazole in recurrent vulvovaginal candidiasis. NEJM Evidence 2022;1(8). EVIDoa2100055.

48. Sobel JD, Chaim W, Nagappan V, et al. Treatment of vaginitis caused by Candida glabrata: use of topical boric acid and flucytosine. Am J Obstet Gynecol 2003; 189(5):1297–300.

49. Shann S, Wilson J. Treatment of Candida glabrata using topical amphotericin B and flucytosine. Sex Transm Infect. Jun 2003;79(3):265–6.

50. White DJ, Habib AR, Vanthuyne A, et al. Combined topical flucytosine and amphotericin B for refractory vaginal Candida glabrata infections. Sex Transm Infect 2001;77(3):212–3.

51. Iavazzo C, Gkegkes ID, Zarkada IM, et al. Boric acid for recurrent vulvovaginal candidiasis: the clinical evidence. J Womens Health (Larchmt) 2011;20(8): 1245–55.

52. Muhleisen AL, Herbst-Kralovetz MM. Menopause and the vaginal microbiome. Maturitas 2016;91:42–50.

53. Shardell M, Gravitt PE, Burke AE, et al. Association of vaginal microbiota with signs and symptoms of the genitourinary syndrome of menopause across reproductive stages. J Gerontol A Biol Sci Med Sci 2021;76(9):1542–50.

54. Martin DH, Zozaya M, Lillis RA, et al. Unique vaginal microbiota that includes an unknown Mycoplasma-like organism is associated with Trichomonas vaginalis infection. J Infect Dis 2013;207(12):1922–31.

55. Hirt RP, Sherrard J. Trichomonas vaginalis origins, molecular pathobiology and clinical considerations. Curr Opin Infect Dis 2015;28(1):72–9.

56. Brotman RM, Bradford LL, Conrad M, et al. Association between Trichomonas vaginalis and vaginal bacterial community composition among reproductive-age women. Sex Transm Dis 2012;39(10):807–12.

57. Nye MB, Schwebke JR, Body BA. Comparison of APTIMA Trichomonas vaginalis transcription-mediated amplification to wet mount microscopy, culture, and polymerase chain reaction for diagnosis of trichomoniasis in men and women. Am J Obstet Gynecol 2009;200(2):188.e1–7.

58. Andrea SB, Chapin KC. Comparison of Aptima Trichomonas vaginalis transcription-mediated amplification assay and BD affirm VPIII for detection of T. vaginalis in symptomatic women: performance parameters and epidemiological implications. J Clin Microbiol 2011;49(3):866–9.

59. Seña AC, Bachmann LH, Hobbs MM. Persistent and recurrent Trichomonas vaginalis infections: epidemiology, treatment and management considerations. Expert Rev Anti Infect Ther 2014;12(6):673–85.

60. Sobel JD, Reichman O, Misra D, et al. Prognosis and treatment of desquamative inflammatory vaginitis. Obstet Gynecol 2011;117(4):850–5.

61. Reichman O, Sobel J. Desquamative inflammatory vaginitis. Best Pract Res Clin Obstet Gynaecol 2014;28(7):1042–50.

62. The 2020 genitourinary syndrome of menopause position statement of The North American Menopause Society. Menopause 2020;27(9):976–92.

63. van de Wijgert J, Verwijs MC. Lactobacilli-containing vaginal probiotics to cure or prevent bacterial or fungal vaginal dysbiosis: a systematic review and recommendations for future trial designs. Bjog 2020;127(2):287–99.
64. Ngugi BM, Hemmerling A, Bukusi EA, et al. Effects of bacterial vaginosis-associated bacteria and sexual intercourse on vaginal colonization with the probiotic Lactobacillus crispatus CTV-05. Sex Transm Dis 2011;38(11):1020–7.

Prevention of Postoperative Surgical Site Infection Following Cesarean Delivery

Maureen S. Hamel, MD, Methodius Tuuli, MD, MPH, MBA*

KEYWORDS

- Cesarean delivery • Wound infection • Infection prevention • Postpartum infection
- Postoperative infection • Obstetrics

KEY POINTS

- Surgical-site infections are a significant complication of cesarean delivery.
- Preoperative skin antisepsis, prophylactic antibiotics, spontaneous placental removal, closure of the subcutaneous tissue, and skin closure with suture are all interventions proven to reduce rates of surgical site infection after cesarean delivery.
- Combinations of interventions into care bundles have also been proven to be effective at reducing infection after cesarean delivery.

BACKGROUND

Cesarean delivery is the most common major surgical procedure performed among birthing persons in the United States. In 2020, 31.8% (1.1 million) of the 3.6 million births in the United States were delivered via cesarean section.[1] With all surgery comes the risk of complications, specifically surgical site infection (SSI). In fact, the strongest risk factor for postpartum infection is cesarean delivery.[2] Depending upon the source, estimates of the rate of SSI following cesarean delivery vary widely and range from as low as 2% to 3% to as high as 15% to 16%.[3–8] Risk factors are well known and include prior cesarean delivery, obesity, diabetes (pregestational and gestational), hypertensive disorders of pregnancy, multiple gestations, preterm premature rupture of membranes, prolonged membrane rupture, intrapartum delivery and intrapartum chorioamnionitis.[4,7,9]

SSI after cesarean delivery poses a significant burden to the patient, not only postpartum and caring for the neonate but also, in many circumstances, caring for other children or household members. Moreover, infections result in increased pain, office visits, and in many cases, hospitalizations that may result in additional procedures.

Department of Obstetrics and Gynecology, 101 Dudley Street, Providence, RI 02905-2499, USA
* Corresponding author.
E-mail address: mtuuli@wihri.org

Obstet Gynecol Clin N Am 50 (2023) 327–338
https://doi.org/10.1016/j.ogc.2023.02.012
0889-8545/23/© 2023 Elsevier Inc. All rights reserved.

In addition to the high patient burden, surgical-site infections increase health care resource utilization and costs. One study estimated the increased hospital cost from surgical-site infection after cesarean to be as high as $2852–$3956.[10]

Despite significant advances in preventive measures, infections remain a significant complication of cesarean delivery.[11] The purpose of this article is to review evidence-based practices for SSI prevention following cesarean delivery.

PREOPERATIVE SKIN ANTISEPSIS

It is well established that skin flora are important pathogenic contributors to SSI and as such, preoperative skin cleansing is a demonstrated avenue to decrease SSI.[3] The 2 most common antiseptic solutions used preoperatively are chlorhexidine and povidone-iodine. Perioperative skin cleansing with each of these solutions, alone and in combination, has been explored in multiple randomized trials with conflicting results.[12–14] In 2015, Ngai and others explored the preoperative application of povidone iodine versus chlorhexidine versus the sequential application of both solutions in a randomized controlled trial with 1,404 participants. While the overall rate of SSI in the study was low at 4.3%, rates of SSI were similar between groups: povidone-iodine 4.6% versus chlorhexidine 4.5% versus sequential application 3.9% ($P = .85$).[12] In 2016, Tuuli and others published another randomized trial of 1,147 participants comparing preoperative chlorhexidine with preoperative iodine. In this study, chlorhexidine-alcohol demonstrated superior efficacy with a decreased rate of wound infection in the chlorhexidine group as compared to the iodine group (RR 0.55; 95% CI 0.34, 0.90).[13] Soon thereafter, in 2017, Springel published a third randomized trial with 932 participants randomized to preoperative chlorhexidine-alcohol versus povidone-iodine-alcohol and again found similar rates of infection between groups (4.6% vs 5.5%; $P = .55$).[14]

In 2019, a systemic review and meta-analysis found that chlorhexidine reduced the rate of surgical site infection over povideine-iodine-based solutions (RR 0.72; 95% CI 0.52, 0.98).[15] Then, in 2020, Cochrane published a systemic review by Hadiati and others that included 13 randomized trials with a total of 6,938 participants. The authors concluded that when compared to povidone iodine, preoperative skin cleansing with chlorhexidine is likely slightly more effective at reducing SSI. While it is clear that perioperative skin cleansing with either solution is effective at reducing SSI following cesarean delivery, the evidence suggests a slight advantage with chlorhexidine.[3,14,15] The Centers for Disease Control and Prevention does not specify the type of preoperative skin cleanser but notes it should be alcohol-based unless contraindicated.[16]

HAIR REMOVAL VIA CLIPPING VERSUS RAZOR REMOVAL

While there is a paucity of data specifically addressing hair removal prior to cesarean delivery, there are data in the surgical literature that can be extrapolated to hair removal at the time of cesarean delivery. Razors are known to have an increased risk of skin abrasion which may contribute to wound infection. In 2021, an updated systemic review published by Tanner demonstrated that when compared with hair clipping, shaving was associated with an increased risk of wound infection (RR 1.64, 95% CI 1.16, 2.33).[17] As such, the use of clippers for hair removal when necessary is encouraged over razor for hair removal.

PREOPERATIVE VAGINAL ANTISEPSIS

In addition to skin cleansing, research has also focused on preoperative vaginal cleansing before cesarean delivery. Bacteria are present in the vagina naturally;

however, at the time of cesarean delivery there is opportunity for these organisms to seed the uterus and surgical wound resulting in postoperative SSI. Both chlorhexidine (low concentration solutions) and povidone-iodine have been investigated as solutions for vaginal cleansing in randomized trials as well as systemic reviews, and results have been mixed. In early randomized trials published by Starr and colleagues in 2005 and Haas and colleagues in 2010 each with over 300 participants, vaginal preparation was compared to no vaginal preparation. Starr and colleagues demonstrated a statistically significant reduction in postoperative endometritis (7% vs 14.5%, $P < .05$) but not wound infection or postoperative fever.[18,19] Haas and colleagues used a composite of infectious morbidity as the primary outcome and were unable to demonstrate a statistically significant difference between the vaginal preparation group and the control group. A critique of these early trials and others is the primary outcome tended to be endometritis but not wound infection and a large proportion of patients enrolled were nonlaboring patients.[18]

A meta-analysis in 2017 including 16 trials and data from 4,837 patients found that among laboring patients or patients with ruptured membranes, that preoperative vaginal antisepsis was associated with a reduced risk of fever and endometritis but not SSI (RR 0.74, 95% CI 0.53, 1.05). The majority of trials in the meta-analysis used povidone-iodine as the vaginal antiseptic solution.[20] In 2018, a secondary analysis of the C-SOAP trial evaluated the rate of superficial or deep SSI in laboring patients from institutions with and without protocols for vaginal preparation with antiseptic solution prior to cesarean delivery. Among 523 parturients delivered at institutions with vaginal preparation protocols, there was no significant difference in superficial or deep SSI when compared with 1,490 parturients delivered at institutions without such protocols (5.5% vs 4.1%; OR 1.38, 95% CI 0.87, 2.17).[21]

In 2020, the Cochrane Database published a revised systemic review evaluating the impact of vaginal preparation with antiseptic solution before cesarean delivery on postoperative infections. Evaluating results from 18 trials with data from 6385 patients, the authors concluded that the risk of postoperative wound infection is likely reduced by vaginal preparation with antiseptic solutions prior to cesarean delivery (RR 0.62, 95% CI 0.50, 0.77). Subgroup analyses suggested that the impact was larger among laboring parturients and was present regardless of the type of vaginal preparation used (iodine or chlorhexidine).[22] As such, preoperative vaginal preparation with iodine or chlorhexidine solutions should be considered prior to CD. Studies demonstrating the superiority of one formulation over the other are lacking. At this time, povidone-iodine is approved for vaginal use and chlorhexidine (low alcohol concentrations) is off-label.

PREOPERATIVE ANTIBIOTICS
Antibiotics Versus No Antibiotic

The utility and efficacy of preoperative antibiotics at cesarean delivery are well established. Antibiotic administration versus no antibiotics at the time of cesarean delivery has been studied in multiple randomized trials. A Cochrane review and meta-analysis first published in 1995, subsequently updated in 2010 and again in 2014, assessed the effect of prophylactic antibiotics compared with none on infectious morbidity in patients undergoing cesarean delivery. Ninety-five studies including data from over 15,000 parturients were included in the analyses. The authors found that prophylactic antibiotic administration in patients undergoing cesarean delivery significantly reduces the incidence of SSI by 60% (RR 0.40, 95% CI 0.35, 0.46).[23]

Single Dose Versus Broad Spectrum/Multi-Dose

Once chemoprophylaxis with first generations cephalosporin was well established, investigators pondered whether extended spectrum single-dose antibiotics[24] or multidose regimens such as ampicillin, gentamycin, and metronidazole[25] would reduce rates of infection even further. None of the randomized trials comparing standard cephalosporin regimens to broader coverage demonstrated superior outcomes with broader coverage. Thus, first-generation cephalosporin is considered the antibiotic of choice or a single-dose combination of aminoglycoside and clindamycin when severe allergies are documented.[26]

Adjunctive Azithromycin

In recent years, evidence has demonstrated that adjunctive azithromycin can further reduce the risk of SSI after cesarean delivery. In 2016 a multicenter randomized trial (C/SOAP) of 2013 patients explored adding azithromycin to standard preoperative antibiotic prophylaxis in patients undergoing nonelective cesarean delivery and its impact on postoperative infection. Patients were randomly assigned to intravenous azithromycin or placebo. The primary outcome was a composite of endometritis, wound infection, or other infection within 6 weeks after delivery. The authors found that azithromycin resulted in a lower rate of the primary outcome as compared to placebo 6.1% versus 12.0% (RR 0.51, 95% CI 0.38, 0.68). Statistically significant differences were also noted in the rate of endometritis and wound infection with lower rates in the intervention group: 3.8% vs 6.1% ($P = .02$) and 2.4 vs 6.6% ($P < .001$), respectively. There were no significant differences between groups with regard to adverse neonatal outcomes.[27] As such, adjunctive azithromycin is recommended for women undergoing nonelective cesarean delivery.[26]

Antibiotics Administration Prior to Skin Incision Versus After Cord Clamping

Timing of antibiotic administration has also been extensively studied. Administration prior to skin incision has been compared to after cord clamping and prior to skin incision is clearly superior at reducing SSI.[28–30] A meta-analysis including these trials demonstrated preoperative administration within 60 minutes of skin incision significantly reduces infectious morbidity when compared to administration at cord clamping (RR 0.5, 95% CI 0.33, 0.78). There was no increased risk of neonatal outcomes demonstrated. While the difference in SSI specifically was not significant (RR 0.6, 95% CI 0.3, 1.21), there was still a trend toward lower risk.[31] Additionally, a retrospective cohort study of more than 9,000 cesarean deliveries explored the rate of infectious morbidity before and after hospital guidelines were changed to advise the administration of antibiotics prior to skin incision at cesarean. The researchers found statistically significantly lower rates of wound infection with preincision administration of antibiotics as compared to administration at cord clamping: 2.5% versus 3.6% (OR 0.69, 95% CI 0.54, 0.88).[32] A subsequent systematic review including 18 randomized trials further strengthened support for preincision antibiotics demonstrating patients receiving antibiotics prior to skin incision had reduced rates of infectious morbidity and wound infection (RR 0.72, 95% CI 0.56, 0.92 and RR 0.57, 95% CI 0.40, 0.82 respectively) when compared to patients that received antibiotics at cord clamping. Again, the risks for neonatal adverse outcomes were not different between groups.[33]

SUPPLEMENTAL OXYGEN

Data from the general surgical literature, specifically in colorectal surgery, have demonstrated an association between high-dose supplemental oxygen and reduced rates of SSI.[34,35] Supplemental oxygen to reduce postoperative SSI following cesarean delivery has been explored in at least 3 randomized trials. All 3 trials randomly assigned patients to receive high-concentration or low-concentration oxygen via mask during cesarean delivery and 1 to 2 hours afterward. None of the trials demonstrated a reduction in SSI among cesarean delivery patients receiving high-dose oxygen supplementation. As such, this supplemental oxygen is not recommended as a preventative intervention at cesarean delivery.[36–38]

PLACENTAL REMOVAL

Multiple studies have investigated the method of placental removal (spontaneous or manual) at the time of cesarean delivery and the impact on postpartum infection. Several trials have found an association between manual placental removal and postpartum endometritis and infectious morbidity.[39–43] A randomized prospective trial including 333 participants comparing manual versus spontaneous placental delivery demonstrated a decreased rate of postoperative infection in the spontaneous delivery group (15% vs 27%, RR 0.6; 95% CI 0.4, 0.9).[41] In 2008, a Cochrane published a systemic review that explored methods of placental delivery at the time of cesarean included 15 trials and data from 4694 patients. The authors concluded that manual removal was associated with increased risk of postpartum endometritis (RR 1.64; 95 CI 1.42, 1.90).[44] While the effect of placental delivery technique on surgical site inspection was not specifically explored, given the association between SSI and endometritis, spontaneous placental removal is recommended.

GLOVE CHANGE

Glove change has been associated with lower rates of surgical-site infection in colorectal surgery.[45] This has also been investigated at the time of cesarean delivery. It is hypothesized that changing gloves intraoperatively may prevent wound infection by reducing the contamination of the wound with commensal flora from the vagina. A recent meta-analysis including 7 randomized trials (1948 patients) demonstrated that glove change during cesarean delivery, was associated with a significantly lower incidence of wound infection (RR 0.41, 95% CI 0.26, 0.65) but not endometritis (RR 0.96, 95% CI 0.78, 1.20). In a subgroup analysis of this data, the intervention seemed to be effective only if performed after delivery of the placenta.[46] Larger randomized trials are needed to fully explore whether glove change at cesarean delivery should be universally recommended.

CLOSURE OF SUBCUTANEOUS TISSUE AND DRAIN PLACEMENT

Multiple studies have explored subcutaneous tissue closure at the time of cesarean delivery. A meta-analysis of randomized trials in 2002 investigated the impact of the closure of the subcutaneous tissue with regard to tissue thickness. While the closure was not associated with a reduced risk of wound infections specifically (RR 0.42; 95% CI 0.65, 1.49), when the subcutaneous thickness was greater than 2 cm, there was a decrease in the rate of a composite of wound complications (RR 0.66; 95% CI 0.48, 0.91).[47] A subsequent Cochrane Review also demonstrated that closure of the subcuticular space reduced composite morbidity that included wound infection (RR 0.68; 95% CI 0.52, 0.88).[48] As such, closure of the subcutaneous tissue is recommended with the thickness exceeds 2 cm.

Drain placement within the subcutaneous tissue has also been explored as this space represents a potential space for seroma or hematoma to form, which could increase the risk of infection. Studies to date show that drain placement in the subcutaneous space is not beneficial in reducing postoperative SSI[49–51]

SKIN CLOSURE

Skin closure has been extensively explored in over 24 randomized trials, 4 meta-analyses and a Cochrane review.[52,53] Suture versus staple has been the most comparison but trials have also investigated the type of suture (monofilament vs multifilament) as well as suture versus glue. A randomized trial including 107 nonlaboring women undergoing scheduled cesarean compared glue (Dermabond; Ethicon, Somerville NJ) to monofilament suture for skin closure. The authors found similar results between groups with regards to surgical time, patient satisfaction, patient satisfaction, SSI, or wound disruption; however, these were scheduled cases and not laboring or emergent during which the risks for SSI are higher.[54]

Another randomized trial compared suture type: monofilament versus multifilament suture. The study included 550 patients undergoing nonemergent cesarean delivery with a primary outcome of a composite that included SSI, wound separation, hematoma, or seroma. Monofilament suture was associated with a decreased rate of wound complications 8.8% versus 14.4% (RR 0.61, p5% CI 0.37, 0.99).[55]

The question regarding suture versus staple closure was recently explored in a meta-analysis of 14 studies published in August 2022. The authors found that suture closure decreased composite wound complications by over 50% (RR0.47, 95% CI 0.28, 0.87). This finding persisted when stratified by obesity (RR 0.51, 95% CI 0.34, 0.75). No differences in cosmesis, patient pain, or patient satisfaction were observed.[53] Given these findings, there is strong evidence to recommend suture closure over staples and likely some added benefit to monofilament over multifilament suture. Currently, there is not enough evidence or data to make recommendations on the use of suture versus glue.

SILVER-IMPREGNATED DRESSING

Silver impregnated dressings have demonstrated some promise in reducing SSI. However, at this time, there is a paucity of data regarding the use of silver-impregnated dressing at cesarean delivery. Two recent studies evaluated the use of silver-impregnated dressings at the time of cesarean delivery; one was a randomized controlled trial and the other was a prospective cohort study. Neither study demonstrated a statistically significant difference in SSI between the intervention and control groups.[56,57]

NEGATIVE PRESSURE WOUND THERAPY

Negative pressure wound therapy (NPWT), also known as vacuum-assisted wound closure, was first approved by the FDA in 1995. This type of closure device uses negative pressure to remove fluid and exudate and as such reduces edema. It also thought to results increase blood flow at the incision site and promote the growth of granulation tissue. While NPWT was initially designed for the treatment of wounds, in 2010 it was approved for prophylactic treatment. In 2016, a meta-analysis of 10 randomized trials explored the use prophylactic use of NPWT for closed incisions. Analyzing data from 1311 incisions in 1089 patients, NPWT resulted in a statistically significant reduction in wound infection when compared to standard surgical dressing (RR 0.54, 95% CI 0.33, 0.89). This meta-analysis did not include any trials investigating NPWT for cesarean delivery incisions.[58]

Two subsequent systemic reviews and meta-analyses were published assessing the effect of prophylactic NPWT after cesarean delivery. The first, by Smid and others from 2017 included 5 randomized controlled trials and 5 cohort studies and explored prophylactic NPWT versus standard dressing after cesarean among obese patients. No difference was observed in the primary outcome which was a composite of wound complication that included SSI, cellulitis, seroma, hematoma, wound disruption, or dehiscence: 16.8% in the NPWT group as compared to 17.8% in the standard dressing group (RR 0.97, 95% CI 0.63, 1.49).[59]

In 2018, Yu and others published another systematic review and meta-analysis; this study included 6 randomized controlled trials and 3 cohort studies assessing the effect of prophylactic NPWT after cesarean delivery on SSI and wound complications. The authors found that when compared with a standard surgical dressing, NPWT after cesarean resulted in a lower risk of SSI (RR 0.45, 95% CI 0.31, 0.66).[60] The conflicting results of these 2 systemic reviews and meta-analyses are not surprising given the small sample sizes and heterogeneity of the included trials with regards to inclusion criteria and types of NPWT. The authors of both papers concluded larger definitive trials are needed to better delineate the role of NPWT in the prevention of SSI after cesarean delivery.

Three subsequent randomized trials have compared the use of prophylactic NPWT versus standard dressing on SSI in obese women undergoing cesarean delivery. Tuuli and colleagues conducted a multi-center randomized trial that assigned obese participants undergoing planned or unplanned cesarean delivery to receive NPWT or standard dressing immediately after incision closure. The primary outcome was SSI. While recruitment was planned for 2850 participants, enrollment was stopped after the enrollment of 1624 when a planned interim analysis demonstrated futility for the primary outcome and an increase in adverse events in the NPWT group. SSI did not differ between the 2 groups: 3.6% in the NPWT group and 3.4% in the standard dressing group (difference 0.36%, 95% CI -1.46%, 2.19%). The only difference the researchers found was in the rate of adverse skin reactions which occurred more frequently in the NPWT group, 7% of participants vs 0.6% of participants in the standard dressing group (difference 6.95%; 95% CI 1.86, 12.03%).[61]

Hyldig and colleagues also published a multi-center randomized trial comparing NPWT with standard dressing after cesarean delivery. This study included 876 obese patients undergoing planned or unplanned cesarean delivery and the primary outcome was SSI requiring antibiotic treatment within the first 30 days after delivery. In this study, the authors did find a statistically significant reduction in SSI among participants in the NPWT group (4.6% compared to 9.2% in the standard dressing group; RR 0.5, 95% CI 0.3–.84). When adjusted for BMI and other possible confounders, results remained significant.[62]

More recently Gillespie and colleagues conducted a multicenter trial in which 2035 patients with prepregnancy body mass index of 30 or greater undergoing elective or semi-urgent cesarean section were randomized before the cesarean procedure to closed incision NPWT (n = 1017) or standard dressing (n = 1018).[63] The primary outcome was cumulative incidence of SSI. In the primary intention to treat analysis, SSI occurred in 75 (7.4%) women treated with closed incision NPWT and in 99 (9.7%) women with a standard dressing a difference that was not statistically significant (risk ratio 0.76, 95% confidence interval 0.57–1.01). Blistering occurred more frequently in the NPWT group (4.0% vs 2.3%; risk ratio 1.72, 1.04–2.85; P = .03).

In conclusion, NPWT devices are costly and the data regarding their efficacy are predominantly show no difference in SSI. Thus, routine use of NPWT to prevent SSI after cesarean is not recommended.

EVIDENCE-BASED BUNDLES

Bundles are a group of evidence-based practices that organizations, typically a hospital or other health care entity, will implement with the goal improving a quality metric such as SSI. While these strategies do not necessarily lend themselves to randomized trials, preimplementation, and postimplementation analyses are common. Several such studies have been published in the obstetric literature addressing SSI after cesarean delivery with favorable results.[64–68] In 2017 a systemic review and meta-analysis of 14 preintervention and postintervention studies, Carter and colleagues demonstrated significantly lower rates of SSI after evidence-based bundle initiation when compared to baseline rates: 2% compared to 6.2% (RR 0.33, 95% CI 0.25, 0.43). It appears that the combination of interventions into a bundle has the potential to result in even further reductions in rates of SSI than anticipated by the individual components alone. However, there was significant heterogeneity between studies and differences in bundle contents, and it is difficult to determine which bundle components are additive, synergistic, or neutral. The authors concluded that despite limitations of heterogeneity and unclear quality of some primary studies, results of this meta-analysis suggest evidence-based bundles are a promising intervention to reduce the risk of surgical site infection among women undergoing cesarean delivery.[69]

SUMMARY

The strongest risk factor for postpartum infection is cesarean delivery. Numerous interventions including preoperative skin antisepsis, prophylactic antibiotic administration, spontaneous placental removal, closure of the subcutaneous tissue, and skin closure with suture have demonstrated reductions in surgical site infection. There is also data to support that when these interventions are combined into bundles, rates decrease even further. As rates continue to improve, research demonstrating effective interventions will become more challenging. Low baseline infection rates mean that interventions aimed at further reducing infection rates have a higher bar to clear; new interventions must be investigated in well-designed studies powered to detect smaller differences. Indeed, as noted earlier, interventions that have plausibility and proven benefit in other subspecialties such as supplemental oxygen, glove change, silver-impregnated dressings, and NPWT have proven ineffective in the setting of cesarean delivery, or data are conflicting. It is possible that the proposed interventions are truly ineffective, or studies may simply be underpowered. Now, more than ever, well-designed randomized trials are critical to identify effective interventions to improve care and reduce morbidity, particularly SSI for patients undergoing cesarean delivery.

CLINICS CARE POINTS

- Evidence-based interventions for prevention of surgical site infections after cesarean include: preoperative skin antisepsis, prophylactic antibiotics, spontaneous placental removal, closure of the subcutaneous tissue if 2 cm or greater, and skin closure with monofilament suture.

- Interventions not shown to be effective include: oxygen supplementation, prophylactic negative pressure wound therapy, subctaneous drains, and silver impregnated dressing.

DISCLOSURES

The authors report no conflict of interest.

REFERENCES

1. Osterman MJK, Hamilton BE, Martin JA, et al. Births: Final data for 2020. NVSR 2022;70(17):1–50.
2. Gibbs RS. Clinical risk factors for puerperal infection. Obstet Gynecol 1980;55(5 Suppl):178S–84S.
3. Hadiati DR, Hakimi M, Nurdiati DS, et al. Skin preparation for preventing infection following cesarean section. Cochrane Database Syst Rev 2020 Jun 25;6(6): CD007452.
4. Kawakita T, Landy HJ. Surgical site infections after cesarean delivery: epidemiology, prevention and treatment. Matern Health Neonatol Perinatol 2017;3:12.
5. Olsen MA, Butler AM, Willers DM, et al. Risk factors for surgical site infection after low transverse cesarean section. Infect Control Hosp Epidemiol 2008;29(6): 477–84.
6. Opoien HK, Valbo A, Grinde-Andersen A, et al. Post-cesarean surgical site infections according to CDC standards: rates and risk factors. A prospective cohort study. Acta Obstet Gynecol Scand 2007;86(9):1097–102.
7. Schneid-Kofman N, Sheiner E, Levy A, et al. Risk factors for wound infection following cesarean deliveries. Int J Gynaecol Obstet 2005;90(1):10–5.
8. Tran TS, Jamulitrat S, Chongsuvivatwong V, et al. Risk factors for postcesarean surgical site infection. Obstet Gynecol 2000;95(3):367–71.
9. Krieger Y, Walfisch A, Sheiner E. Surgical site infection following cesarean deliveries: trends and risk factors. J Matern Fetal Neonatal Med 2017;30(1):8–12.
10. Olsen MA, Butler AM, Willers DM, et al. Attributable costs of surgical site infection and endometritis after low transverse cesarean delivery. Infect Control Hosp Epidemiol 2010;31(3):276–82.
11. Conroy K, Koenig AF, Yu YH, et al. Infectious morbidity after cesarean delivery: 10 strategies to reduce risk. Rev Obstet Gynecol 2012;5(2):69–77.
12. Ngai IM, Van Arsdale A, Govindappagari S, et al. Skin preparation for prevention of surgical site infection after cesarean delivery: A randomized controlled Trial. Obstet Gynecol 2015;126(6):1251–7.
13. Tuuli MG, Liu J, Stout MJ, et al. A randomized trial comparing skin antiseptic agents at cesarean delivery. N Engl J Med 2016;374(7):647–55.
14. Springel EH, Wang XY, Sarfoh VM, et al. A randomized open-labor controlled trial of chlorhexidine-alcohol versus povidone-iondine for cesarean antisepsis: the CAPICA trial. Am J Obstet Gynecol 2017;217(4):463.e1–8.
15. Tolcher MC, Whitman MD, El-Nasha SA, et al. Chlorhexidine-alcohol compared with povidone-iodine preoperative skin antisepsis for cesarean delivery: A systemic review and meta-anlysis. Am J Perinatol 2019;36(2):118–23.
16. Berrios-Torres SI, Umscheid CA, Bratzler DW, et al. Centers for disease control and prevention guideline for the prevention of surgical site infection. JAMA Surg 2017;152(8):784–91.
17. Tanner J, Melen K. Preoperative hair removal to reduce surgical site infection. Cochrane Database Sys Rev 2021 Aug 26;8(8):CD004122.
18. Starr RV, Zurawski J, Imail M. Preoperative vaginal preparation with povidone-iodine and risk of postcesarean endometritis. Obstet Gynecol 2005;105(5 Pt 1): 1024–9.
19. Haas DM, Pazouki F, Smith RR, et al. Vaginal cleansing before cesarean delivery to reduce postoperative infectious morbidity: a randomized, controlled trial. Am J Obstet Gynecol 2010;202(3):310.e1–6.

20. Caissutti C, Saccone G, Zullo F, et al. Vaginal cleansing before cesarean delivery: a systemic review and meta-analysis. Obstet Gynecol 2017;130(3):527–34.
21. La Rosa M, Jauk V, Saade G, et al. Institutional protocols for vaginal preparation with antiseptic solution and surgical site infection rate in women undergoing cesarean delivery during labor. Obstet Gynecol 2018 Aug;132(2):371–6.
22. Haas DM, Morgan S, Contreras K, et al. Vaginal preparation with antiseptic solution before cesarean section for preventing postoperative infections. Cochrane Database Syst Rev 2020;4(4):CD007892.
23. Smalll FM, Grivell RM. Antibiotic prophylaxis versus no prophylaxis for preventing infection after cesarean section. Cochrane Database Sys Rev 2014;2014(10):CD007482.
24. Ziogos E, Tsiodras S, Matalliotakis I, et al. Ampicillin/sulbactam versus cefuroxime as antimicrobial prophylaxis for cesarean delivery; a randomized study. BMC Infect Dis 2010;10:341.
25. Alekwe LO, Kuti O, Orji EO, et al. Comparison of ceftriaxone versus triple drug regimen in the prevention of cesarean section infectious morbidities. J Matern Fetal Neonatal Med 2008;21(9):638–42.
26. Committee on Practice Bulletins-Obstetrics. ACOG practice bulletin No. 199: Use of prophylactic antibiotics in labor and delivery. Obstet Gynecol 2018;132(3):e103–19.
27. Tita ATN, Szychowski JM, Boggess K, et al. Adjunctive azithromycin prophylaxis for cesarean delivery. N Eng J Med 2016;375(13):1231–41.
28. Sullivan SA, Smith T, Chang E, et al. Administration of cefazolin prior to skin incision is superior to cefazolin at cord clamping in preventing post-cesarean infectious morbidity: a randomized controlled trial. Am J Obstet Gynecol 2007;196(5):455.e1–5.
29. Thigpen BD, Hood WA, Chauhan S, et al. Timing of prophylactic antibiotic administration in the uninfected laboring gravida: a randomized clinical trial. Am J Obstet Gynecol 2005;192(6):1864–71.
30. Wax JR, Hersey K, Philput C, et al. Single dose cefazolin prophylaxis postcesarean infections: before vs after cord clamping. J Matern Fetal Med 1997;6(1):61–5.
31. Costantine MM, Rahman M, Ghulmiyah L, et al. Timing of perioperative antibiotics for cesarean delivery: a metaanalysis. Am J Obstet Gynecol 2008;199(3):301.e1–6.
32. Owens SM, Brozanski BS, Meyn LA, et al. Antimicrobial prophylaxis for cesarean delivery before skin incision. Obstet Gynecol 2009;114(3):573–9.
33. Bollig C, Nothacker M, Lehane C, et al. Prophylactic antibiotics before cord clamping in cesarean delivery: a systemic review. Acta Obstet Gynecol Scand 2018;97(5):521–35.
34. Belda FJ, Aguilera L, Garcia de la Asuncion J, et al. Supplemental perioperative oxygen and the risk of surgical wound infection: A randomized controlled trial. JAMA 2005;294(16):2035–42.
35. Greif R, Acka O, Horn EP, et al, Outcomes Research Group. Supplemental perioperative oxygen to reduce the incidence of surgical wound infection. N Eng J Med 2000;342(3):161–7.
36. Duggal N, Poddatorri V, Noroozkhani S, et al. Perioperative oxygen supplementation and surgical site infection after cesarean delivery: A randomized trial. Obstet Gynecol 2013;122(1):79–84.
37. Gardella C, Goltra LB, Laschansky E, et al. High-concentration supplemental perioperative oxygen to reduce the incidence of postcesarean surgical site infection: a randomized controlled trial. Obstet Gynecol 2008;112(3):545–52.

38. Scifres CM, Leighton BL, Fogertey PJ, et al. Supplemental oxygen for the prevention of postcesarean infectious morbidity: a randomized controlled trial. Am J Obstet Gynecol 2011;205(3):267.e1–9.
39. Atkinson MW, Owen J, Wren A, et al. The effect of manual removal of the placenta on post-cesarean endometritis. Obstet Gynecol 1996;87(1):99–102.
40. Chandra P, Schiavelo HJ, Kluge JE, et al. Manual removal of the placenta and postcesarean endometritis. J Reprod Med 2002;47(2):101–6.
41. Lasley DS, Eblen A, Yancey MK, et al. The effect of placental removal method on the incidence of postcesarean infections. Am J Obstet Gynecol 1997;176(6): 1250–4.
42. Magann EF, Washburne JF, Harris RL, et al. Infectious morbidity, operative blood loss, and length of the operative procedure after cesarean delivery by method of placental removal and site of uterine repair. J Am Coll Surg 1995;181(6):517–20.
43. McCurdy CM, Magann EF, McCurdy CJ, et al. The effect of placental management at cesarean delivery on operative blood loss. Am J Obstet Gynecol 1992; 167(5):1363–7.
44. Anorly RI, Maholwana B, Hofimeyr GJ. Methods of delivering the placenta at cesarean section. Cochrane Database Syst Rev 2008;3:CD004737.
45. Cima R, Dankbar E, Lovely J, et al. Colorectal surgery surgical site infection reduction program: a national surgical quality improvement program–driven multidisciplinary single-institution experience. J Am Coll Surg 2013;216(1):23–33.
46. Narice BF, Almeida JR, Farrell T, et al. Impact of changing gloves during cesarean section on postoperative infective complications: A systematic review and meta-analysis. Acta Obstet Gynecol Scand 2021;100(9):1581–94.
47. Chelmow D, Huang E, Strohbehn K. Closure of the subcutaneous dead space and wound disruption after cesarean delivery. J Matern Fetal Neonatal Med 2002;11(6):403–8.
48. Anderson ER, Gates S. Techniques and materials for closure of the abdominal wall in caesarean section. Cochrane Database Syst Rev 2004 Oct 18;2004(4): CD004663.
49. Hellums EK, Lin MG, Ransey PS. Prophylactic subcutaneous drainage for prevention of wound complications after cesarean delivery- a meta-analysis. Am J Obstet Gynecol 2007;197(3):229–35.
50. Magann EF, Chauhan SP, RodtsPalenik S, et al. Subcutaneous stitch closure versus subcutaneous drain to prevent wound disruption after cesarean delivery: a randomized clinical trial. Am J Obstet Gynecol 2002;186(6):1119–23.
51. Ramsey PS, White AM, Guinn DA, et al. Subcutaneous tissue re-approximation alone or in combination with drain in obese women undergoing cesarean delivery. Obstet Gynecol 2005;105(5 Pt 1):967–73.
52. Dahlke JD, Mendez-Figueroa H, Maggio L, et al. The Case for Standardizing Cesarean Delivery Technique: Seeing the Forest for the Trees. Obstet Gynecol 2020; 136(5):972–80.
53. Mackeen AD, Sullivan MV, Schuster M, et al. Suture compared with staples for skin closure after cesarean delivery: A systemic review and meta-analysis. Obstet Gynecol 2022;140(2):293–303.
54. Daykan Y, Sharon-Weiner M, Pasternak Y, et al. Skin closure at cesarean delivery, glue vs subcuticular sutures: a randomized controlled trial. Am J Obstet Gynecol 2017;216(4):406.e1–5.
55. Buresch AM, Van Arsdale A, Ferzli M, et al. Comparison of subcuticular suture type for skin closure after cesarean delivery: a randomized controlled trial. Obstet Gynecol 2017;130(3):521–6.

56. Connery SA, Yankowitz J, Odibo L, et al. Effect of using silver nylon dressings to prevent superficial surgical site infection after cesarean delivery: a randomized clinical trial. Am J Obstet Gynecol 2019;221(1):57.e1–7.

57. Goodman JR, Durazo-Arvizu R, Nashif S, et al. Preventing cesarean section wound complications: use of a silver-impregnated antimicrobial occlusive dressing. J Wound Care 2022;31(Sup7):S5–14.

58. Hyldig N, Birke-Sorensen H, Kruse M, et al. Meta-analysis of negative pressure wound therapy for closed surgical incisions. Br J Surg 2016;103(5):477 86.

59. Smld MC, Dotters-Katz SK, Grace M, et al. Prophylactic negative pressure wound therapy for obese women after cesarean delivery: A systemic review and meta-analysis. Obstet Gynecol 2017;130(5):969–78.

60. Yu L, Kronen RJ, Simon Mlis LE, et al. Prophylactic negative pressure wound therapy after cesarean is associated with reduced risk of surgical site infection: a systemic review and meta-analysis. Am J Obstet Gynecol 2018;218(2):200–10.

61. Tuuli MG, Lie J, Tita ATN, et al. Effect of prophylactic negative pressure wound therapy vs standard wound dressing on surgical-site infection in obese women after cesarean delivery: a randomized clinical trial. JAMA 2020;324(12):1180–9.

62. Hyldig N, Vinter CA, Kruse M, et al. Prophylactic incisional negative pressure wound therapy reduces the risk of surgical site infection after cesarean section in obese women: A pragmatic randomized clinical trial. BJOG 2019;126(5):628–35.

63. Gillespie BM, Webster J, Ellwood D, et al. Closed incision negative pressure wound therapy versus standard dressings in obese women undergoing caesarean section: multicentre parallel group randomised controlled trial. BMJ 2021;373:n893.

64. Corcoran S, Jackson V, Coulter-Smith S, et al. Surgical site infection after cesarean section: implementing 3 changes to improve the quality of patient care. Am J Infect Control 2013;41(12):1258–63.

65. Kawakita T, Iqbal SN, Landy HJ, et al. Reducing cesarean delivery surgical site infections: a resident-driven quality initiative. Obstet Gynecol 2019;133(2):282–8.

66. Pritchard A, Donohue K, Hyland T, et al. Reducing cesarean delivery surgical site infection: successful implementation of a bundle of care. Obstet Gynecol 2016;127(suppl 1):7S.

67. Riley MM, Suda D, Tabsh K, et al. Reduction of surgical site infections in low transverse cesarean section at a university hospital. Am J Infect Control 2012;40(9):820–5.

68. Salim R, Braverman M, Berkovic I, et al. Effect of interventions in reducing the rate of infection after cesarean delivery. Am J Infect Control 2011;39(10):e73–8.

69. Carter EB, Temming LA, Fowler S, et al. Evidence-based bundles and cesarean delivery surgical site infections: A systemic-review and meta-analysis. Obstet Gynecol 2017;130(4):735–46.

Human Papillomavirus Vaccine
The Cancer Prevention Moonshot

Kelsey Petrie, MD, MPH[a], Alex Wells, MD, MBs[a],
Linda O. Eckert, MD[b],*

KEYWORDS

- HPV vaccine • Vaccine equity • Cervical cancer • HPV virus • Oncogenic virus

KEY POINTS

- Cervical cancer strikes more than 600,000 individuals with a cervix a year.
- The human papillomavirus (HPV) vaccine, when given at the 9 to 14 years recommended age range, can prevent 90% of cervical cancer.
- The HPV vaccine can also prevent most of the throat, anal, vulvar, and vaginal cancers when administered at the targeted age range.
- HPV vaccination remains underused in the United States as a robust cancer prevention tool.
- Global HPV vaccine supply is currently restricted, and many lower income and middle-income countries do not have access to this cancer prevention tool, despite having the highest burden of cervical cancer.

BACKGROUND

The approval of the HPV vaccine in 2006 ushered in an unprecedented era as a tool to prevent cervical cancer, in addition to other human papillomavirus (HPV)–caused malignancies. Given the public attention of the Cancer Moonshot efforts, here is a "moonshot" at our fingertips. In the case of the HPV vaccine, we claim both that the Moonshot has landed, but that for many, it remains a far away journey.

Burden of Disease

HPV is the most common sexually transmitted infection (STI) worldwide. It is a DNA virus causing mostly asymptomatic infections, with incidence peaking among those

The authors have no financial disclosures or intellectual conflicts of interest.
[a] Department of Obstetrics & Gynecology, University of Washington School of Medicine, 1959 Pacific Avenue, Box 356460, Seattle, WA 98195, USA; [b] Department of Obstetrics & Gynecology, Adjunct Department of Global Health, University of Washington School of Medicine, 1959 Pacific Avenue, Box 356460, Seattle, WA 98195, USA
* Corresponding author.
E-mail address: eckert@uw.edu

Obstet Gynecol Clin N Am 50 (2023) 339–348
https://doi.org/10.1016/j.ogc.2023.02.006
0889-8545/23/© 2023 Elsevier Inc. All rights reserved.

obgyn.theclinics.com

at younger ages, 90% of whom will clear the infection within 24 months without intervention.[1] There are more than 150 strains of the HPV virus, and persistence of replicating virus with a carcinogenic strain can lead to precancerous and cancerous lesions.[1,2] The time from initial infection with HPV to an invasive HPV-associated cancer in those with persistent disease is on average 15 to 20 years and dependent on HPV strain, individual immunological status, other coinfections, and tobacco use, among others.[2] The cancers associated with HPV include cervical, penile, vulvar, vaginal, anal, and oropharyngeal carcinoma.[1,2] In the United States approximately 37,000 new cases of HPV attributable cancers occur annually.[1] Although HPV infections can cause a variety of cancers, for this review the authors focus on cervical cancer, as it has the largest proportion of global morbidity and mortality of the HPV-associated cancers.[2] The authors use the terms "female," "women," and "girls" to describe genetic females with the understanding that not everyone with a cervix may identify as a female, woman, or girl.

Cervical cancer is the fourth most common cancer among females worldwide.[2] Globally, 91% of HPV-related cancers in females are cervical cancers, and most of the cases are attributable to infection with an oncogenic HPV strain[2]; these include HPV 16 (50% of cervical cancer cases); HPV 18 (20%); and HPV 31, 33, 45, 52, and 58 (19% combined).[2–4] In 2020, there were just more than 600,000 new cases of and 340,000 deaths from cervical cancer globally.[2] This HPV-associated cancer clearly has an immense impact—not just for those contracting the cancer—but also far beyond. When a woman dies, the impact on her children and those in her family is detrimental and life altering, not to mention the loss in our societal fabric.

An important distinction in the discussion of cervical cancer is that between the 2 major subtypes, adenocarcinoma and squamous cell carcinoma. Most of the cervical cancers (70%–75%) are squamous cell; adenocarcinoma is less common (25%). High-grade cervical dysplasia is a risk factor for both. Squamous cell cervical carcinoma is more commonly associated with HPV 16 (60%) than with HPV 18 (13%). Adenocarcinoma, on the other hand, is more commonly associated with HPV 18 (37%) than HPV 16 (36%). Although squamous cell carcinoma remains the most common cervical cancer type, adenocarcinoma is increasing in incidence, is less readily identified on routine PAP smear, develops at a younger age than squamous carcinoma, and may have a worse prognosis.[5,6]

In the United States, the incidence of not only adenocarcinoma but also stage IV cervical cancer at diagnosis is increasing. A recent study found a rate of increase in diagnosis of stage IV cervical cancer at diagnosis of 1.3% a year in the last 18 years, with a 2.9% increase in adenocarcinoma of the cervix; this is certainly alarming given the 5-year survival rate of 17%. This study also found that in the United States, black women have disproportionately high rates of stage IV cervical cancer at diagnosis (1.55 times the rate of white women). In addition, it found the population with the highest rate of increase to be young white women (ages 40–44 years) in the Southern United States, with a rate of increase of 4.5% a year. White women also have higher rates of absent guideline-based screening, and white teenagers have the lowest rates of HPV vaccination.[7] Inequities exist in the United States surrounding later stage diagnosis, increasing incidence, and guideline-based screening.

Difference in HPV infection and cervical cancer rates exist on a global scale as well. Although worldwide the prevalence of HPV infection among those with normal cytology is approximately 12%, in Sub-Saharan African it is 24%.[8–10] Eighty-four percent of cervical cancer cases worldwide are from resource-limited regions. Among females in these regions, cervical cancer is the second most common type of cancer and the third most common cause of cancer mortality. In Africa and Central America, it is the leading cause of cancer-related mortality. The mortality rates also vary significantly with a rate of less than 2 per 100,000 in higher income countries compared with 28 per 100,000 in lower income countries, an 18-fold increase; this is due to a lack of widespread HPV vaccination, a lack of screening and treatment of cervical precancer, and absence of treatment options in many low-resource settings.[2,8,9]

Further, human immunodeficiency virus (HIV) infection intensifies HPV carcinogenesis. Females with HIV are at an increased risk of progression to high-grade dysplasia and subsequent cervical cancer.[10] Among females with HIV, there is 6 times the risk of cervical cancer. South and Eastern Africa are the most effected; in Eastern African nearly 27% of females with cervical cancer also live with HIV. In Southern Africa this number is nearly 64%.[11]

The Human Papillpmavirus Vaccine

HPV was found to be an oncogenic virus in the 1980s; after this discovery there was a relatively rapid production of a quadrivalent HPV vaccine first authorized for use in the United States in 2006 for HPV 6, 11, 16, and 18. Soon after, the bivalent vaccine was released in 2007 for HPV 16 and 18, followed by the nonavalent vaccine in 2014 covering the most HPV strains yet (HPV 6, 11, 16, 18, 31, 33, 45, 52, and 58).[2] The goal with each is to administer before onset of sexual activity and thus exposure to HPV for maximum efficacy.[1,2] All 3 vaccines use recombinant DNA technology, none contain live virus, and therefore they cannot transmit virus. HPV protection comes from neutralizing antibodies to the major HPV viral coat protein, L1. This purified structural L1 protein self-assembles to form HPV type–specific viral-like particles against high-risk HPV types included in the specific vaccine that are highly immunogenic. These vaccine-induced immunoglobulin G antibodies then reach the site of a natural HPV infection to neutralize virus.[2]

All of the HPV vaccines initially were approved with a 3-dose vaccination schedule. After evidence of noninferiority with a 2-dose vaccination schedule, this was approved for each vaccine in individuals 9 to 14 years of age.[2] The World Health Organization (WHO) Strategic Advisory Group of Experts on Immunization (SAGE) released a statement in early 2022 stating that a single dose of the HPV vaccine garners similar protection to a 2-dose schedule.[12] Although this has not been adopted in the United States, it may in time as the evidence emerges. Currently in the United States, a 2-dose regimen (vaccination at 0, 6–12 months) is recommended for those who receive the first dose before the age of 15 years, and a 3-dose regimen (vaccination at 0, 1–2, and 6 months) is recommended for those who receive the first dose after the age of 15 or with immunocompromising conditions.[1]

With either dosing schedule, the HPV vaccine is highly efficacious. It has the potential to prevent 90% of HPV attributable cancers and is 99% efficacious against HPV 16 and 18 if administered before exposure.[1,10] The immune response to the vaccine is much higher than with natural infection. As the vaccine nears 2 decades on the market, there are now excellent longevity data, and it does not seem a booster is needed.[10] A single case of cervical cancer can be prevented by vaccinating 70 females. In addition, among HIV-positive patients seroconversion against HPV has reliably been observed underscoring the vaccines potential to alleviate disparities in HPV infection and subsequent cervical cancer.[2,10]

The current WHO recommendations are to prioritize HPV vaccination of females ages 9 to 14 years before the onset of sexually active, with the goal of reaching 90% full vaccination by age 15 years by the year 2030 to eliminate cervical cancer as a public health issue.[2,10] The most recent WHO position statement notes that gender-neutral vaccination globally is less cost-effective than focusing vaccination efforts on girls and thus specifically prioritizes females.[2] In the United States, HPV vaccination is recommended for 11- to 12-year-old girls as well as 13- to 26-year-old girls who have not been vaccinated or did not complete the series with a similar goal of vaccination before initiation of sexual activity and exposure to HPV, although the vaccine can be given as early as age 9 years.[1] In addition, routine vaccination of 11- to 12-year-old boys or those aged 13 to 26 years not previously vaccinated or who have not received all recommended doses is recommended in the United States.[1] Some adults aged 27 to 45 years who are not fully vaccinated may benefit from the vaccine and can have individual decision-making discussions with their health care provider about the HPV vaccine.[1]

Human Papillomavirus Vaccine Uptake and Distribution

The HPV vaccine has the enormous potential to prevent cervical (and other) HPV-associated cancers. In the United States, the benefit of the availability of the HPV vaccine in terms of HPV infection rates is clear. In a recent analysis comparing HPV rates between females born in the 1980s and those born in the 1990s, HPV infection rates decreased from 12.5% to 5.6%, respectively. Even more encouraging, the rates of HPV 16 and 18 infection, the most oncogenic strains, decreased from 15.2% to 3.3% over the decade.[13] Since being approved in the United States in 2006, HPV vaccination coverage among adolescents has increased over time; as of 2021 nearly 77% of adolescents in the United States had received at least 1 dose, with 62% being up-to-date.[14] Yet despite estimates that initiation of HPV vaccination programs could, over the next 100 years, prevent 60 million cases of and 45 million deaths from cervical cancer, to date just 125 countries or 64% have initiated an HPV vaccine program within their national immunization program.[2] What has affected uptake and distribution of this life-saving vaccine on a global scale?

As previously mentioned, the WHO recommended the vaccine be given to all females ages 9 to 14 years in 2009. National vaccination campaigns, however, require money and infrastructure. The formal WHO recommendation did allow lower income countries to receive some funding and access to the vaccine through Gavi, an international public private aid organization. Gavi provides support to the 54 countries with the lowest annual gross domestic product and was able to secure a price of $4.55 for the HPV vaccine, significantly less expensive than the more than $100 it initially cost in the United States.[15] Yet, as of 2022, most of the Gavi-supported countries have yet to launch a national HPV program.[15] Further, most middle-income countries that do not qualify for Gavi funding, but that do not have the national public health funding for a new HPV national vaccination program, remain without HPV vaccine programs. The new evidence from SAGE that a single-dose regimen is acceptable is hoped to mitigate barriers around cost and resources bolstering national vaccination efforts.[12]

In the United States, despite being a wealthy nation with funds and infrastructure, the cancer-preventing HPV vaccine certainly was not met with immediate and rapid uptake. In the first year after the HPV vaccine was recommended in the United States, 25% of females received it. By 2015 63% had received at least 1 dose, and in 2021 77% of females (and 74% of males) had received 1 dose.[14,16] Although this has translated to decreasing HPV infections and has continued to increase with public health efforts, it is certainly not the 90% WHO benchmark. Reasons parents in the United States cite for choosing to not vaccinate their children include feeling the vaccine is not necessary, lack of provider recommendation, and not being a school requirement.[17] Sexual stigma around HPV as an STI has also been identified as a barrier.[18] Cost has also been cited as a reason; in the United States for those who qualify under the age of 18 years the vaccination is paid for by Vaccines For Children, a federally funded income-based program through the CDC.[1] For those who do not quality for this assistance, the cost is just more than $250 for each dose, with the actual cost being insurance based and variable.[19]

Several HPV vaccine delivery models have been associated with rapid and high rates of uptake. Countries in high- and low-income settings that use school-based vaccination have achieved high coverage. In Australia, the national HPV vaccination program was initiated as a school-based program in 2007; this led to a national rate of 83% for vaccination initiation soon after and 70% for completion with increasing coverage in recent years. Such a program has been said to have a "normative influence" that is convenient for parents.[20] Similarly, in Rwanda starting in 2011 the 3-dose course was given free of charge to females in grade 6, with 93% coverage nationwide. This was after significant planning efforts centered on reaching females in and out of schools, partnering between the Ministry of Health and Education, and using community health workers. There were coordinated speeches by health-care professionals, clergy, and government officials including the First Lady promoting the HPV vaccine, and teachers were trained to discuss the vaccine with their students before the roll-out.[21]

In the United States, where school-based HPV vaccine is rarely used, high coverage has been achieved when delivering the HPV vaccine in a culturally accepted manner. One example is the Navajo Area Indian Health Service Unit in Chinle Arizona, which achieved a nearly 83% HPV vaccination rate among teenage girls (compared with 50% in Arizona among females age 13–17 years and 47% of American Indian and Alaska natives nationwide of the same age); this was accomplished by deliberate efforts by the Service unit to "weave HPV vaccination into Navajo culture by connecting it to coming-of-age ceremonies that observe transition into adulthood" and including traditional healers.[22] These efforts have been exceedingly effective and show that culturally appropriate planning, infrastructure, and support can lead to high HPV vaccination rates.

Cost-Effectiveness

The cost-effectiveness of the HPV vaccination has been well studied in the United States and globally. In the United States, the economic costs of HPV-related warts and cervical disease is estimated to be $4 billion annually.[23,24] In a 2008 analysis, a simplified incidence-based model was used to examine the health and economic effects of implementing HPV vaccination in 12-year-old girls. The study aimed to address the question, "What is the cost per QALY gained by adding vaccination of 12-year-old girls to existing cervical cancer screening practices in the United States?". The quality-adjusted life-year (QALY) is a generic health measure of disease burden. QALY attempts to combine the morbidity and mortality of a disease or health condition into a single number and estimate how many quality months or years a person may gain as a result of a particular treatment. The study examined HPV-related health outcomes including cervical cancer, cervical intraepithelial neoplasia (CIN) 1 to 3, genital warts, some anal cancer, vaginal vulvar cancer, and oropharyngeal cancer. Cervical cancer treatment costs averted were calculated using the number of cervical cancer cases prevented by vaccination and the estimated cost per case of cervical cancer. The number of QALYs saved by vaccination was calculated using the age-specific number of cervical cancer cases averted by the vaccine and the estimated number of QALYs lost per case of cervical cancer. The study found that cost per QALY gained by adding routine vaccination of 12-year-old girls to current cervical cancer screening ranged from $3906 to $14723.[25] Given the cost per QALY gained is less than $50,000,

HPV vaccination is cost-effective in the United States. A similar study out of Canada examining HPV vaccination in 12-year-old females also found HPV vaccination to be cost-effective. The Canadian study estimates $18672 to $31687 per QALY gained and approximately 390 to 633 prevented cervical cancer cases.[26]

The cost-effectiveness of HPV vaccination has also been well studied globally. In a 2014 study, 179 countries were examined using the Papilloma Rapid Interface for Modeling and Economics (PRIME) model. The PRIME model estimates the health and economic effect of vaccination in terms of age-dependent incidence of cervical cancer and mortality in direct proportion to vaccine efficacy against HPV 16 and 18. Results of the study were validated by comparison with 17 other published studies and all 72 published GAVI-eligible countries. The study found that HPV vaccination was very cost-effective in 156 (87%) out of 179 countries.[27] Another study published in 2021 was a meta-regression analysis looking at cost-effectiveness of HPV vaccination in 195 countries. The study analyzed previously published cost-effectiveness analyses. Factors were analyzed at the country, intervention, and method level and to predict incremental cost-effectiveness ratios (ICERs). The mean predicted ICER was 4217 United States Dollars (USD) per disability-adjusted life-years (DALY, an estimate of overall disease burden considering healthy years of life lost secondary to a given disease), averted globally. ICER was lowest in sub-Saharan Africa and South Asia with a mean of $706 USD per DALY averted and $489 per DALY averted across 5 countries.[28] These numbers confirm that use of the HPV vaccine in sub-Saharan Africa and in South Asia is extremely cost-effective and a prudent investment well worthy of competing for scarce public health dollars.

Equity

As with most of the health care today, HPV and cervical cancer are not exempt from issues of health equity, access, and commercialism. In May of 2018, the WHO issued a call to action to eliminate cervical cancer as a public health problem. The WHO has created the cervical cancer elimination initiative and adopted the global strategy for cervical cancer elimination in August of 2020. Vaccination is one of the WHO's 3 key pillars in achieving cervical cancer eradication. As previously mentioned, the vaccination target set by the WHO call for 90% of girls to be fully vaccinated by the age of 15 years by the year 2030.[29] As of 2020 less than 25% of low-income countries had implemented HPV vaccination compared with 85% of high-income countries.[30]

There are several factors that have made expanding access to vaccination challenging, among which is the global HPV vaccine shortage. In the 2020 UNICEF Human Papillomavirus Vaccine: Supply and Demand Update, UNICEF breaks down some of the factors influencing global shortage. At the time of their analysis, there were only 2 manufacturers the WHO has qualified for HPV vaccines, Merck and GlaskoSmithKline. The analysis estimated that in 2020 the global market would require 44.5 million doses of HPV vaccine, up significantly from the 30 to 35 million doses per year from 2010 to 2016.[15] Factors that have contributed to the increase in demand include the introduction of vaccine to India and China, increase in gender neutral immunization policies, and the WHO call to end cervical cancer that has stressed the need for equitable access to HPV vaccine.[31] With only 2 manufacturers, supply has struggled to keep up with demand, and it is predicted this shortage will continue for the near future.

The COVID 19 pandemic has also had a substantial negative impact on efforts at expanding HPV vaccination. Much of the infrastructure used for vaccination globally uses locations where communities gather such as schools, community centers, and places of worship. Closures and limitations on gathering have resulted in millions of girls missing out on vaccination. The pandemic also caused a massive reallocation of public health resources away from routine immunization and toward the global pandemic. According to a study by UNICEF and WHO, the COVID-19 pandemic resulted in 23 million children missing out on scheduled vaccination and 1.6 million girls missing out on HPV vaccinations in 2020.[32] In a recent study, the long-term effects of missed HPV vaccines in the United States during the COVID pandemic is estimated evaluating vaccine uptake data from January 2018 to August 2020 and applies it to 4 different scenarios for post-COVID vaccination catch up. With the most optimistic vaccine recovery there are 130,000 additional cases of genital warts, 22,000 cases of CIN1, and 48,000 cases of CIN2/3 over the next 100 years. More than 50% of the cases of genital warts, CIN 1, and CIN2/3 would occur in the next 25 years. The scenarios also project an associated increase in cervical cancer cases. In the most optimistic projection of these increases, there are 2882 additional cases of cervical cancer, with 66% occurring in the first 50 years.[33]

LITTLE KNOWN FACTS ABOUT HUMAN PAPILLOMAVIRUS AND HUMAN PAPILLOMAVIRUS VACCINATION

As we continue to learn more about HPV, there have been some unexpected discoveries. For instance, an association between coinfection with HPV and Trichomonas vaginalis and an increase in the risk of CIN have been demonstrated. More specifically, the study found that although coinfection with Candida or Gardnerella with HPV did not have as association with CIN, T vaginalis coinfection was associated with both more oncogenic HPV strains and an increase in the risk of CIN 1 by an odds ratio (OR) of 1.8 and CIN 2/3 by an OR of 1.71.[34]

Male circumcision has also been researched in association with HPV. Circumcision has been well studied in sub-Saharan Africa with HIV acquisition and transmission, and this research is actively expanding to other STIs. Most of the data show a protective association between male circumcision and risk of HPV infection in both African and European settings.[35] Male circumcision has also been shown to reduce the risk of oncogenic HPV genotypes and cervical cancer.[36]

The Long View

Australia could serve as one of the first examples of what cervical cancer eradication could look like. As previously discussed, Australia was one of the first countries to introduce a national HPV vaccination program in 2007 and did so for a wide age range from 12 to 26 years with a school-based program.[20] Australia has also had a national cervical cancer screening program since 1991, which has resulted in an approximately 50% decrease in cervical cancer incidence.[37] In a modeling study in 2019, it was estimated that by 2028 the incidence of cervical cancer in Australia will be fewer than 4 new cases per 100,000 women and less than 1 per 100,000 by 2066. Further, by 2034 the cervical cancer mortality is projected to decrease to less than 1 death per 100,000 women.[38] Australia is thus a clear example of the immense potential impact of prioritization of HPV vaccine uptake with the goal of eradication of cervical cancers by a multitude of public health entities. Eradication, or near eradication, is possible.

SUMMARY

The HPV vaccine is an unprecedented tool to prevent HPV-mediated cancers, of which, cervical cancer has the largest global burden of disease. The cost of the HPV vaccine, inequitable access, delivery challenges, and a global supply shortage, combined with the stigma of talking about and preventing a "below the belt" cancer, have kept it from becoming the cancer prevention miracle that it is. However, with the

WHO's call to eliminate cervical cancer elevating the global discussion about this vaccine, as well as efforts to increase HPV vaccine supply, in so facilitating lower pricing and improving access, and creative determination to increase its use, we can look forward to more individuals able to access this Cancer Moonshot.

CLINICS CARE POINTS

- HPV is a common virus that is sexually transmitted and has 14 subtypes that cause cancer.
- Of the HPV virus types, HPV 16 and HPV 18 combined account for 70% of cervical cancer.
- All HPV vaccines offer protection against HPV 16 and HPV 18 when the vaccine is given before exposure to these viruses.
- One HPV vaccine, the nonavalent HPV vaccine, in addition to protecting against HPV types 16 and 18, also offers protection against HPV types 31, 33, 45, 52, and 58. This vaccine protects against 90% of cervical cancer.
- Because the HPV vaccine works to prevent infection (versus eliminate infection once it is present), the best time to give the HPV vaccine is in the 9 to 14 years age range.
- When given to individuals younger than 15 years, 2 doses are approved, given 6 to 12 months apart, although the WHO also has stated that 1 dose of HPV vaccine may be considered in individuals 20 years of age or younger (instead of 2 doses).
- For individuals 15 years old or older, or for individuals who are immunocompromised, 3 doses of the HPV vaccine are needed, with the second dose 1 to 2 months after the first dose and the third dose 4 months after the second.

REFERENCES

1. Control CfD. Human Papillomavirus. 2021. Available at: https://www.cdc.gov/hpv/index.html. Accessed September 22, 2023.
2. Organization WH. Human papillomavirus vaccines: WHO position paper, December 2022. 2022. Available at: https://www.who.int/publications/i/item/who-wer9750. Accessed January 19, 2023.
3. de Sanjose S, Quint WG, Alemany L, et al. Human papillomavirus genotype attribution in invasive cervical cancer: a retrospective cross-sectional worldwide study. Lancet Oncol 2010;11(11):1048–56.
4. Serrano B, Alemany L, Tous S, et al. Potential impact of a nine-valent vaccine in human papillomavirus related cervical disease. Infect Agent Cancer 2012; 7(1):38.
5. Li N, Franceschi S, Howell-Jones R, et al. Human papillomavirus type distribution in 30,848 invasive cervical cancers worldwide: Variation by geographical region, histological type and year of publication. Int J Cancer 2011;128(4):927–35.
6. Castanon A, Landy R, Sasieni PD. Is cervical screening preventing adenocarcinoma and adenosquamous carcinoma of the cervix? Int J Cancer 2016;139(5): 1040–5.
7. Francoeur AA, Liao CI, Caesar MA, et al. The increasing incidence of stage IV cervical cancer in the USA: what factors are related? Int J Gynecol Cancer 2022;32:1115–22.
8. Torre LA, Bray F, Siegel RL, et al. Global cancer statistics, 2012. CA Cancer J Clin 2015;65(2):87–108.

9. Sung H, Ferlay J, Siegel RL, et al. Global Cancer Statistics 2020: GLOBOCAN estimates of incidence and mortality worldwide for 36 cancers in 185 countries. CA Cancer J Clin 2021;71(3):209–49.

10. sageexecsec@who.int WHOEa. Human papillomavirus vaccines: WHO position paper, May 2017-Recommendations. Vaccine 2017;35(43):5753–5.

11. Stelzle D, Tanaka LF, Lee KK, et al. Estimates of the global burden of cervical cancer associated with HIV. Lancet Glob Health 2021;9(2):e161–9.

12. Organization WH. One-dose Human Papillomavirus (HPV) vaccine offers solid protection against cervical cancer. 2022. Available at: https://www.who.int/news/item/11-04-2022-one-dose-human-papillomavirus-(hpv)-vaccine-offers-solid-protection-against-cervical-cancer. Accessed September 22, 2022.

13. Shahmoradi Z, Damgacioglu H, Montealegre J, et al. Prevalence of human papillomavirus infection among women born in the 1990s vs the 1980s and Association With HPV Vaccination in the US. JAMA Health Forum 2022;3(8):e222706.

14. Prevention CfDCa. . National Vaccination Coverage Among Adolescents Aged 13-17 Years – National Immunization Survey -Teen, United States, 2021. 2022. Available at: https://www.cdc.gov/mmwr/volumes/71/wr/mm7135a1.htm. Accessed January 22, 2023.

15. Gavi. Human Papillomavirus Vaccine Support. 2018. Available at: https://www.gavi.org/types-support/vaccine-support/human-papillomavirus. Accessed January 22, 2023.

16. Pingali C, Yankey D, Elam-Evans LD, et al. National, regional, state, and selected local area vaccination coverage among adolescents aged 13-17 years - United States, 2020. MMWR Morb Mortal Wkly Rep 2021;70(35):1183–90.

17. Hirth JM, Fuchs EL, Chang M, et al. Variations in reason for intention not to vaccinate across time, region, and by race/ethnicity, NIS-Teen (2008-2016). Vaccine 2019;37(4):595–601.

18. Peterson CE, Silva A, Goben AH, et al. Stigma and cervical cancer prevention: a scoping review of the U.S. literature. Prev Med 2021;153:106849.

19. Gardasil. Information about Gardasil. Manufacturer's website. Available at: https://www.gardasil9.com/adults/cost/. Accessed January 22, 2023.

20. Skinner R., Davies C., Brotherton J., Australia's national HPV vaccination program. In. HPV World: The Newsletter on HPV. no 114. Available at: https://www.hpvworld.com/articles/australia-s-national-hpv-vaccination-program/. Accessed February 23, 2023.

21. Binagwaho A, Wagner CM, Gatera M, et al. Achieving high coverage in Rwanda's national human papillomavirus vaccination programme. Bull World Health Organ 2012;90(8):623–8.

22. Christensen A. Navajo Nation Home to Region's Highest HPV Vaccination Rate. 2018. Available at: https://cancercenter.arizona.edu/news/2018/04/navajo-nation-home-region's-highest-hpv-vaccination-rate. Accessed January 22, 2023.

23. Chesson HW, Blandford JM, Gift TL, et al. The estimated direct medical cost of sexually transmitted diseases among American youth, 2000. Perspect Sex Reprod Health 2004;36(1):11–9.

24. Insinga RP, Dasbach EJ, Elbasha EH. Assessing the annual economic burden of preventing and treating anogenital human papillomavirus-related disease in the US: analytic framework and review of the literature. Pharmacoeconomics 2005; 23(11):1107–22.

25. Chesson HW, Ekwueme DU, Saraiya M, et al. Cost-effectiveness of human papillomavirus vaccination in the United States. Emerg Infect Dis 2008;14(2):244–51.

26. Anonychuk AM, Bauch CT, Merid MF, et al. A cost-utility analysis of cervical cancer vaccination in preadolescent Canadian females. BMC Public Health 2009; 9:401.

27. Jit M, Brisson M, Portnoy A, et al. Cost-effectiveness of female human papillomavirus vaccination in 179 countries: a PRIME modelling study. Lancet Glob Health 2014;2(7):e406–14.

28. Rosettie KL, Joffe JN, Sparks GW, et al. Cost-effectiveness of HPV vaccination in 195 countries: A meta-regression analysis. PLoS One 2021;16(12):e0260808.

29. Organization WH. Global strategy to accelerate the elimination of cervical cancer as a public health problem. 2020. https://www.who.int/publications/i/item/97892 40014107. Accessed January 27, 2023.

30. Organization WH. Immunization, Vaccines and Biologicals. Available at: https://www.who.int/teams/immunization-vaccines-and-biologicals. Accessed January 27, 2023.

31. Unicef. Human Papillomavirus Vaccine: Supply and Demand Update. 2022. Available at: https://www.unicef.org/supply/media/5406/file/Human-Papillomavirus-Vaccine-Market-Update-October2020.pdf. Accessed January 27, 2023.

32. Organization WH. WHO UNICEF Immunization Coverage Estimates. 2022. Available at: https://www.who.int/docs/default-source/immunization/immunization-coverage/wuenic_notes.pdf?sfvrsn=88ff590d_6. Accessed January 27, 2023.

33. Daniels V, Saxena K, Roberts C, et al. Impact of reduced human papillomavirus vaccination coverage rates due to COVID-19 in the United States: A model based analysis. Vaccine 2021;39(20):2731–5.

34. Yang M, Li L, Jiang C, et al. Co-infection with trichomonas vaginalis increases the risk of cervical intraepithelial neoplasia grade 2-3 among HPV16 positive female: a large population-based study. BMC Infect Dis 2020;20(1):642.

35. Grund JM, Bryant TS, Jackson I, et al. Association between male circumcision and women's biomedical health outcomes: a systematic review. Lancet Glob Health 2017;5(11):e1113–22.

36. Morris BJ, Hankins CA, Banerjee J, et al. Does male circumcision reduce women's risk of sexually transmitted infections, cervical cancer, and associated conditions? Front Public Health 2019;7:4.

37. Smith M, Canfell K. Impact of the australian national cervical screening program in women of different ages. Med J Aust 2016;205(8):359–64.

38. Hall MT, Simms KT, Lew JB, et al. The projected timeframe until cervical cancer elimination in Australia: a modelling study. Lancet Public Health 2019;4(1): e19–27.

Prevention of Perinatal Hepatitis B Transmission

David M. Higgins, MD, MS[a], Sean T. O'Leary, MD, MPH[a],*

KEYWORDS

- Hepatitis B • Perinatal • Prevention • Vaccination • Postexposure prophylaxis

KEY POINTS

- Hepatitis B virus (HBV) is efficiently transmitted to newborn infants in the perinatal period and can lead to chronic infection, cirrhosis, liver cancer, and death.
- Effective prevention measures to eliminate perinatal HBV transmission are readily available including maternal screening, treatment with antiviral medication, postexposure prophylaxis for newborn infants at risk of acquisition, and universal vaccination at birth.
- Significant gaps remain in the implementation of perinatal HBV transmission prevention measures.
- All clinicians who care for pregnant persons and their newborn infants play a critical role in the successful implementation of perinatal HBV transmission prevention measures.

INTRODUCTION
Nature of the Problem

Hepatitis B virus (HBV) is a viral pathogen transmitted by blood or sexual contact which can be efficiently transmitted to newborn infants in the perinatal period.[1] Without proper identification and postexposure prophylaxis, 70% to 90% of perinatally exposed newborn infants will acquire HBV infection.[1] Up to 90% of those newborn infants infected with HBV will develop chronic infection which can lead to cirrhosis, liver cancer, and death.[2] In response to this threat, a comprehensive strategy to prevent perinatal HBV transmission was introduced in the United States in 1991 and has continued to evolve over the past three decades.[3] Other North American countries have adopted similar national or local perinatal prevention strategies.[4–6] The World Health Organization (WHO) and the United States have initiated strategies to eliminate perinatal HBV transmission as a public health threat by 2030.[7–9]

Effective prevention measures necessary to eliminate perinatal HBV transmission as a public health threat already exist. The cornerstones for the prevention of perinatal

[a] Department of Pediatrics, University of Colorado School of Medicine, Adult and Child Center for Health Outcomes Research and Delivery Science (ACCORDS), University of Colorado/Children's Hospital Colorado, Mailstop F443, 1890 North Revere Court, Aurora, CO 80045, USA
* Corresponding author.
E-mail address: Sean.Oleary@cuanschutz.edu

Obstet Gynecol Clin N Am 50 (2023) 349–361
https://doi.org/10.1016/j.ogc.2023.02.007
0889-8545/23/© 2023 Elsevier Inc. All rights reserved.

HBV transmission include (1) identification of maternal cases through universal screening of pregnant persons for HBV infection and treatment with antiviral medication for pregnant persons with high viral loads, (2) timely postexposure prophylaxis (PEP) of infants born to persons with HBV infection with both HBV vaccine and HBV immune globulin (HBIG), and (3) timely universal vaccination of infants at birth with HBV vaccine as a safeguard to protect infants born to mothers infected with HBV who were not identified.[3] These cornerstones of perinatal HBV transmission prevention have developed and improved over time with advancements in diagnostic tests, maternal HBV treatments, and a better understanding of best practices in screening, PEP, and HBV vaccination.

Despite significant achievements over the past three decades in the identification of HBV surface antigen (HBsAg)-positive pregnant persons, newborn infants appropriately receiving PEP, and rates of HBV vaccination at birth, perinatal transmission of HBV remains a significant public health threat in North America. North American countries remain well below national and international targets for perinatal HBV transmission prevention efforts.[2,5,8] This failure to reach prevention targets in North America disproportionately affects disadvantaged populations who experience a higher burden of HBsAg positivity including pregnant persons who are Asian or Pacific Islanders, non-Hispanic Blacks, born outside of the United States and Canada, or people who are non-English speaking.[10–12]

Although the prevention measures necessary to eliminate perinatal HBV transmission already exist and are readily available in North American countries, considerable improvements in the dissemination and implementation of these prevention measures are necessary to reach the goal of eliminating perinatal HBV transmission. All clinicians who care for pregnant persons and their infants play an integral role in the implementation of these measures. This article summarizes and discusses the evidence, current guidelines, and updates regarding the prevention of perinatal HBV transmission.

Epidemiology

Worldwide, an estimated 1.5 million new infections with HBV occur every year and this is largely driven by perinatal transmission.[13] In 2019, the WHO estimates 296 million people were living with chronic HBV infection worldwide and the HBV infection caused 820,000 deaths.[5] Most of these deaths occur as a result of chronic liver disease or cancer.[5] In 2019, the Centers for Disease Control and Prevention (CDC) estimated there were 20,700 newly acquired HBV infections in the United States.[14] An estimated 880,000 to 1.89 million people in the United States are living with chronic HBV infection, a majority of whom are unaware of their infection.[15,16] The rate of new HBV infections in the United States and the prevalence of chronic HBV have not decreased over the past decade.[15] Non-US born residents account for an estimated 69% of people in the United States living with chronic HBV infection.[15] Of particular concern is the impact of the opioid epidemic which has contributed to a significant proportion of incident HBV cases in the United States, with 35% of new infections associated with injection drug use in 2019.[14] Additionally, the coronavirus disease 2019 (COVID-19) pandemic resulted in significant changes in health-seeking behavior and disruptions in HBV testing and reporting which may have affected surveillance and prevention efforts.[17]

In the United States, approximately 20,000 infants are born to HBsAg-positive persons every year.[12,18] Despite readily available and highly effective prevention measures, approximately 1000 new cases of perinatal HBV infection occur annually in the United States.[19] Perinatal transmission can occur in utero, during the birthing process, or after birth; however, in utero transmission is estimated to account for less than

2% of all cases of perinatal HBV infection.[1] Transmission of HBV in the perinatal period is highly efficient with up to 90% of newborn infants at risk for acquiring the infection if born to a mother who is HBsAg-positive.[1] The risk for perinatal HBV acquisition is greater in newborn infants born to mothers who are HBV e antigen (HBeAg) positive compared with those who are HBeAg negative.[2,20,21] However, maternal HBeAg status is often unknown as it is not generally included in routine screening. Additionally, newborn infants born to mothers with high HBV DNA levels (>200,000 IU/mL) are at an increased risk of infection even with appropriate PEP; however, this increased risk of transmission can be reduced with antiviral therapy.[1,22] Newborn infants are also at greater risk for HBV acquisition if born to mothers who acquire a new HBV infection late in pregnancy, highlighting the need for repeated HBsAg screening at delivery for pregnant persons at high risk of HBV acquisition[2,23] Conversely, breastfeeding is not a significant route of perinatal HBV transmission.[1] In newborn infants who receive appropriate PEP, there is no additional risk of HBV acquisition through breastmilk and these infants can safely breastfeed.[1,23–25]

PREVENTION OF PERINATAL HEPATITIS B VIRUS TRANSMISSION
Prevention Measures

The available measures for the prevention of perinatal HBV transmission are extremely effective. An HBV vaccine that is both safe and effective has been available in the United States since 1992.[26,27] The HBV vaccine alone, when given within 24 hours of birth, is 75% to 95% effective at preventing perinatal HBV transmission.[28] When infants born to HBsAg-positive mothers receive appropriate PEP with HBV vaccine and HBIG within 12 hours of birth, followed by completion of the HBV vaccine series, only 0.7% to 1.1% of infants develop an infection.[2] When maternal antiviral treatment is added to PEP in pregnant persons with high HBV DNA levels, the risk of perinatal HBV transmission is reduced further.[22]

Progress in Prevention Measure Implementation

Significant achievements have been made worldwide toward the elimination of perinatal HBV transmission.[29] These achievements have resulted in the attainment of a global 2020 target of HBsAg prevalence below 1% among children younger than 5 years old.[5] Elimination of perinatal HBV transmission as a public health threat is defined by the WHO as ≤ 0.1% prevalence of HBsAg among children ≤ 5 years old, as well as ≥ 90% coverage with the HBV vaccine birth dose and the complete series of HBV vaccine.[29] Although 98% of the 194 WHO member states had introduced HBV vaccine recommendations for children, only 57% have universal recommendations for a birth dose of HBV vaccine. Additionally, only 11 countries that recommend a universal birth dose of the HBV vaccine have demonstrated an HBsAg seroprevalence of ≤ 0.1% among children ≤ 5 years old.[29] Furthermore, the COVID-19 pandemic contributed to substantial disruptions in perinatal HBV transmission preventive measures worldwide, the effects of which are yet to be fully understood.[5,29]

Considerable progress has also been made in the United States toward the goal of eliminating perinatal HBV transmission since a comprehensive national strategy to prevent perinatal HBV transmission was introduced in 1991.[3] Since the introduction of the HBV vaccination in 1982, the United States has seen a greater than 90% reduction in reported cases of acute HBV infection. However, significant gaps in perinatal transmission prevention measures remain. Using insurance claims data from 2014, one study demonstrated that approximately 88% of commercially insured and 84% of

Medicaid-enrolled pregnant women received HBsAg testing during their pregnancy; however, only 60% of commercially insured and 39.4% of Medicaid-enrolled pregnant women were tested during the first trimester as recommended.[30] A separate study of commercially insured data from 2011 to 2014 demonstrated that only 42% of pregnancies with an associated HBV infection code were linked with appropriate HBV infection care during pregnancy.[31] Although a large managed health care system in California was able to achieve high compliance with HBV DNA testing (93% of HBsAg-positive pregnant women were tested for HBV DNA as recommended), little is known about the rate of testing for HBV DNA in other populations and health systems.[32]

When HBsAg-positive mothers are identified and referred for case management in the United States, 97% of their newborn infants receive PEP within 12 hours of birth and 85% complete the HBV vaccine series.[18] This is in large part due to the efforts of the national Perinatal Hepatitis B Prevention Program (PHBPP), which aims to facilitate timely PEP to infants born to HBsAg-positive pregnant persons, ensure these infants receive the complete HBV vaccine series, and perform recommended postvaccination serologic testing. The PHBPP has achieved great success in managing cases; however, as of 2017, it was estimated that only 53% of the estimated births to HBsAg-positive persons in the United States are identified and referred to the PHBPP.[18] This large gap highlights both the need for vigilance in screening and referral of HBsAg-positive pregnant persons and the universal administration of a timely birth dose of HBV vaccine to prevent transmission in mothers not identified during pregnancy. The CDC has set the following PHBPP targets for 2024: (1) 80% of estimated births to HBsAg-positive mothers will be identified, (2) 98% of identified newborn infants receive PEP, (3) 90% of identified newborn infants receive PEP and complete the HBV vaccine series, (4) and 85% of identified newborn infants receive PversusT.[18]

Despite the availability of a safe and effective vaccine for HBV since 1982 and a universal birth dose recommendation since 1991,[33] among children born during 2015 to 2016, only 75% of newborn infants received a dose of HBV vaccine within 3 days of birth, which was far below the Healthy People 2020 target of 85%.[34] This reason for the gap in HBV birth dose coverage is multifactorial and includes a lack of parental education, inadequate hospital birth dose policies, parental refusal, and a lack of health care provider recommendations.[35–37] Parents requesting non-standard or delayed childhood immunization schedules frequently request HBV vaccine to be delayed.[38] Filling in these significant gaps is critical to the successful elimination of perinatal HBV transmission.

CURRENT EVIDENCE FOR THE PREVENTION OF PERINATAL HEPATITIS B VIRUS TRANSMISSION

The current recommendations reviewed here are consistent with and based on recommendations from the American College of Obstetricians and Gynecologists, Society for Maternal-Fetal Medicine, American Academy of Pediatrics (AAP), Advisory Committee on Immunization Practices (ACIP), American Association for the Study of Liver Disease (AASLD), and the WHO.[2,28,39–42] Although the recommendations from these various advisory groups have evolved and at times differed slightly, the cornerstones of prevention remain (1) identification of maternal cases through universal screening of pregnant persons for HBV infection and treatment with antiviral medication for pregnant persons with high viral loads, (2) timely PEP of infants born to HBsAg-positive persons with both HBV vaccine and HBIG, and (3) timely universal vaccination of infants at birth with HBV vaccine as a safeguard to protect infants born to mothers infected with HBV who were not identified through routine screening.[3]

Identification of Hepatitis B Virus Surface Antigen-Positive Pregnant Persons and Antiviral Treatment of Pregnant Persons with High Viral Loads

Key points of prevention measure

- All pregnant persons should be tested for HBsAg during an early prenatal visit (first trimester) in each pregnancy, regardless of vaccination history, previous testing, or known chronic infection (**Fig. 1**).[2]
- All pregnant persons with an initial negative HBsAg screen who are at high risk for acquisition of HBV (recent or current injection drug use, having had more than one sex partner in the previous 6 months, or an HBsAg-positive sex partner, having been evaluated or treated for a sexually transmitted infection) should be re-screened for HBsAg at time of admission for delivery.[43]
- All pregnant persons not tested prenatally or those with signs of clinical hepatitis should be tested at the time of admission for delivery.[2]
- All pregnant persons who are HBsAg-positive should be referred to their jurisdiction's PHBPP for case management.[2]
- All pregnant persons who are HBsAg-positive should be tested for HBV DNA levels.[2]
- The AASLD recommends antiviral therapy for HBsAg-positive pregnant persons with HBV DNA levels greater than 200,000 IU/ML (7.6 log10 IU/mL).[39]

The recommendations for testing HBV DNA levels in all HBsAg-positive pregnant persons and subsequent antiviral therapy for viral DNA levels greater than 200,000

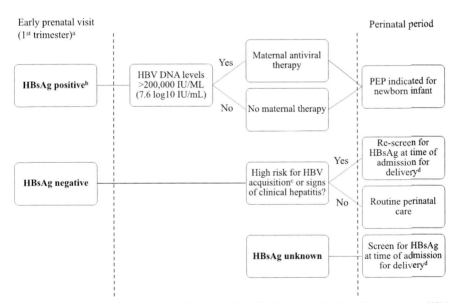

Fig. 1. Prenatal screening for hepatitis B infection. HBsAg, hepatitis B surface antigen; HBV, hepatitis B virus; PEP, post-exposure prophylaxis. [a]All pregnant persons should be tested for HBsAg during an early prenatal visit (1st trimester) in each pregnancy, regardless of vaccination history, previous testing or known chronic infection. [b]All pregnant persons who are HBsAg-positive should be referred to their jurisdiction's PHBPP for case management. [c]Risk for HBV acquisition includes recent or current injection-drug use, having had more than one sex partner in the previous 6 months or an HBsAg-positive sex partner, having been evaluated or treated for a STI. [d]See **Table 1** for PEP recommendations for newborn infants born to mothers with unknown HBsAg status.

IU/ML (7.6 log10 IU/mL) is a new recommendation as of 2018.[2,39] This recommendation from the ACIP and AASLD is based on a growing body of evidence that demonstrates newborn infants are at risk of infection, despite receiving appropriate PEP, if maternal HBV DNA levels remain elevated but this risk can be reduced with antiviral therapy.[2,22,39] A systemic review and meta-analysis of studies concluded there is evidence that antiviral therapy improves HBV suppression and reduces perinatal HBV transmission risk compared with the use of PEP alone.[22] Antiviral therapy, started at 28 to 32 weeks' gestation, has been associated with reduced rates of perinatal HBV transmission.[22] The preferred antiviral agent is tenofovir as it is not associated with resistance and the available data support the safety of tenofovir use in pregnancy.[2] A more detailed review of HBV treatment in pregnancy can be found in guidelines from the AASLD.[39]

Pregnant persons known to be chronically infected with HBV should still have HBsAg testing performed. Documentation of the positive HBsAg result during pregnancy helps with referral programs and ensures all staff involved in the care of the mother and infant at delivery are aware of the mother's HBsAg-positive status so that timely PEP is administered.[2] When pregnant persons are tested for HBsAg at the time of admission for delivery, laboratories may be able to use shortened testing protocols to expedite positive result notification and timely PEP administration.[2]

Postexposure Prophylaxis for all Newborn Infants Born to Hepatitis B Virus Surface Antigen-Positive Mothers

Key points of prevention measure

- All newborn infants born to HBsAg-positive mothers should receive HBV vaccine and HBIG within 12 hours of birth, regardless of newborn infant weight (**Table 1**).[2]
- All infants born to mothers with unknown HBsAg results who have evidence suggestive of maternal HBV infection (positive HBV DNA test, HBeAg-positive, or known chronic infection with HBV) should be managed in the same way as if the mother was HBsAg-positive.[2]
- All infants born to mothers with unknown HBsAg results should receive HBV vaccine within 12 hours while awaiting the results of maternal HBsAg testing which should be performed as soon as possible on admission for delivery. If maternal HBsAg is found to be positive, the newborn infant should receive HBIG as soon as possible but no later than 7 days of life.[2]
- All infants weighing less than 2000 g who are born to mothers with unknown HBsAg results should receive HBV vaccine within 12 hours of life and HBIG at 12 hours of life if the mother's HBsAg status cannot be determined by that time.[2]

The timely administration of PEP to infants at risk for HBV acquisition is critical to the success of this prevention measure. When PEP is delayed, the effectiveness of this intervention decreases substantially.[44] ACIP recommendations from 2018 emphasize the importance of not delaying PEP in cases where the mother's HBsAg status is unknown but there is other clinical concern for risk of maternal HBV.[2] Additionally, in these recommendations, there is an emphasis on clear communication between facilities if newborn infants born to HBsAg-positive or unknown mothers are transferred to a different facility after birth such as a hospital with a higher level of neonatal care to ensure PEP is not delayed.[2] Additionally, all pregnant persons who are HBsAg-positive should receive information on HBV infection, the risk to their infant, the importance of life-saving PEP, completing the HBV vaccination series, and PversusT.[2] In cases where parents refuse the recommendation for PEP, providers should consider seeking intervention through child protective services, given the significant risk of harm to the child.[45]

Table 1
Birth dose of hepatitis B vaccine and/or hepatitis B immune globulin for newborn infants by maternal hepatitis B virus surface antigen status and birthweight

Maternal HBsAg Status	Birthweight	Dose	Timing of Administration After Birth
Positive	≥ 2,000 g	HBV vaccine HBIG[b]	≤ 12 h ≤ 12 h
Unknown[a]		HBV vaccine	≤ 12 h
Negative		HBV vaccine	≤ 24 h
Positive	< 2,000g	HBV vaccine HBIG	≤ 12 h ≤ 12 h
Unknown		HBV vaccine HBIG	≤ 12 h ≤ 12 h
Negative		HBV vaccine	Hospital discharge or age 1 mo (whichever is earlier)

Abbreviations: HBIG, hepatitis B immune globulin; HBsAg, hepatitis B surface antigen; HBV, hepatitis B virus.

[a] Mothers should have blood drawn and tested for HBsAg as soon as possible after admission for delivery; if the mother is found to be HBsAg-positive, the infant should receive HBIG as soon as possible but no later than age 7 d.

[b] HBIG should be administered at a separate anatomic site from vaccine.

Adapted from Schillie S, Vellozzi C, Reingold A, et al. Prevention of Hepatitis B Virus Infection in the United States: Recommendations of the Advisory Committee on Immunization Practices. MMWR Recomm Rep. Jan 12 2018;67(1):1-31.

Universal Vaccination of all Newborn Infants Born to Hepatitis B Virus Surface Antigen-Negative Mothers

Key points of prevention measure

- All medically stable infants weighing ≥ 2,000 g who are born to HBsAg-negative mothers should receive HBV vaccine within 24 hours after birth.[2]
- All infants weighing less than 2000 g who are born to HBsAg-negative mothers should receive HBV vaccine at 1 month of age or at hospital discharge (whichever is first).[2]

The HBV vaccine alone, when given within 24 hours of birth, is 75% to 95% effective at preventing perinatal HBV transmission.[28] The recommendation for the administration of the universal birth dose of HBV vaccine has evolved over time. In 2017, the ACIP rescinded prior permissive language in recommendations that allowed for delaying the HBV vaccine birth dose until after discharge "on a case-by-case basis and only in rare circumstances". The current ACIP recommendations are in line with WHO recommendations to give the birth dose within 24 hours.[28] The timely universal vaccination of all newborns at birth is a safety net for cases where the maternal HBV screening labs were not obtained, misinterpreted, incorrectly transcribed, or falsely negative, which can occur with maternal acquisition of HBV infection in pregnancy after the initial screening.[45]

ADDITIONAL RECOMMENDATIONS
Hepatitis B Virus Vaccination of Pregnant Mothers

- Pregnant individuals who lack documentation of complete HBV vaccination or evidence of past infection should be vaccinated during pregnancy.[46]

In 2018, the reported HBV vaccination coverage rate (≥3 doses) in adults ≥ 19 years of age in the United States was 30.0%.[46] For this reason, as of 2022, the ACIP recommends universal HBV vaccination in adults aged 19 to 59 years (including pregnant persons) who have not been previously vaccinated or have documented evidence of prior HBV infection.[46] This removes the risk factor-based approach previously recommended to determine HBV vaccine eligibility in this age group.[46] Providers should only accept dated records of past HBV vaccination. Pre-vaccination testing, which consists of testing for HBsAg, antibody to HBsAg (anti-HBs), and antibody to HBV core antigen, can be performed in populations with a high rate of previous HBV infection to reduce costs by avoiding complete vaccination of persons who are already immune. However, testing is not a requirement for vaccination and a lack of access to serologic testing should not be a barrier to vaccination of susceptible persons. Vaccination of persons already immune to HBV infection because of previous vaccination or infection has not been shown to increase the risk for adverse events. Providers should vaccinate pregnant persons needing HBV vaccination with Engerix-B, Recombivax HB, or Twinrix as these have been sufficiently studied in pregnancy and found to have a desirable safety profile.[46]

Intrapartum Considerations

- The delivery route should be determined by obstetric indications alone.[2,47]

The evidence for elective cesarean sections to prevent perinatal HBV transmission is poor and data are conflicting. Several studies demonstrate no difference in perinatal transmission among newborn infants delivered by operative or spontaneous vaginal delivery versus cesarean section when infants receive appropriate PEP.[48] Although there have been reports that elective cesarean section may reduce the risk of perinatal HBV transmission, the quality of the evidence is poor.[49] For these reasons, it is recommended that the delivery route be determined by obstetric indications alone.[2,42]

Breastfeeding

- Infants born to HBsAg-positive mothers can safely breastfeed immediately after birth.[50]

When appropriate PEP is given to newborn infants born to HBsAg-positive mothers, studies have demonstrated no difference in rates of infection between breastfed and formula-fed infants.[24] In line with recent AAP recommendations, newborn infants should be encouraged to breastfeed immediately after birth without waiting for the administration of PEP.[50]

Infant Follow-Up

- The full HBV vaccine series should be completed according to the ACIP/CDC recommendations for HBV childhood vaccination. For infants weighing less than 2000 g, the birth dose should not be counted as a part of the full HBV vaccine series out of concern for reduced immunogenicity in these infants. Three additional doses of the vaccine (four doses total) should be administered starting 1 month after birth.[2]
- For all newborn infants born to HBsAg-positive mothers, PversusT for anti-HBs and HBsAg should be performed at 9 to 12 months of age after completion of the HBV vaccine series. HBsAg-negative infants with anti-HBs levels less than 10 mIU/mL should be revaccinated with a single dose of HBV vaccine and receive PversusT 1 to 2 months later. Infants whose anti-HBs remains less than 10 mIU/mL after the revaccination dose should receive two additional revaccination doses of HBV vaccine to complete three doses for the second series, followed by PversusT 1 to 2 months after the final dose.[2]

DISCUSSION

Perinatal HBV transmission is preventable and the effective prevention measures needed to eliminate transmission are readily available. However, the elimination of perinatal HBV transmission relies on the successful implementation of these measures. This starts with all providers who care for pregnant persons and their newborn infants understanding these prevention measure and how to use them. However, whereas knowledge about prevention measures is necessary, knowledge alone is not sufficient for successful implementation. Errors in the delivery of these prevention measures are not rare events. On annual surveys conducted by the Immunization Action Coalition, in one 3-year period covering 1999 to 2002, there were more than 500 reported medical errors regarding perinatal HBV prevention.[51] In a recent survey of obstetricians in California, only 70% routinely advised HBsAg-positive patients to seek specialist evaluation for antiviral treatment and 49% routinely provided them with HBV information.[52] Additionally, increasing trends in vaccine refusal, delay, and hesitancy complicate efforts to increase universal HBV vaccine birth dose coverage.

Universal policies, procedures, and systems that ensure these measures are consistently applied should be developed and tailored to individual health care settings. The electronic health record should be leveraged to successfully implement these types of protocols with standing orders, prompts, and reminders. Clear communication, hand-offs, and documentation between clinicians caring for the mother and those caring for the infant are essential to the successful timely administration of PEP. Finally, all providers who care for pregnant persons and their children should receive education and understand best practices in vaccine communication to improve universal HBV vaccine acceptance at birth.

SUMMARY

Although effective prevention measures including screening, maternal treatment, PEP, and vaccination to prevent perinatal HBV transmission already exist and are readily available in the North American countries, the dissemination and implementation of these measures into practice are critical to the elimination of perinatal HBV transmission. Clinicians who care for pregnant persons and their children must have a clear understanding of these prevention measures and their appropriate use.

CLINICS CARE POINTS

- All pregnant persons should be tested for HBsAg during an early prenatal visit (first trimester) in each pregnancy.
- All pregnant persons with an initial negative HBsAg screen who are at high risk for acquisition of HBV should be re-screened for HBsAg at the time of admission for delivery.
- All pregnant persons who are HBsAg-positive should be tested for HBV DNA levels and treated with antiviral medication for viral DNA levels greater than 200,000 IU/ML (7.6 log10 IU/mL).
- All pregnant persons who are HBsAg-positive should be referred to their jurisdiction's PHBPP for case management.
- All newborn infants born to HBsAg-positive mothers should receive the HBV vaccine and HBIG within 12 hours of birth.
- All medically stable infants weighing $\geq$ 2000 g who are born to HBsAg-negative mothers should receive the HBV vaccine within 24 hours after birth.

- Pregnant persons who lack documentation of complete HBV vaccination or evidence of past infection should be vaccinated during pregnancy.
- Infants born to HBsAg-positive mothers can safely breastfeed immediately after birth.

CONFLICTS OF INTEREST DISCLOSURES (INCLUDES FINANCIAL DISCLOSURES)

D.M. Higgins was supported in part by the Health Resources and Services Administration (HRSA) of the U.S. Department of Health and Human Services (HHS) under grant number D33HP31669. This information or content and conclusions are those of the author and should not be construed as the official position or policy of, nor should any endorsements be inferred by HRSA, HHS, or the US Government. The authors have nothing else to disclose.

REFERENCES

1. Committee on Infectious Diseases American Academy of Pediatrics, Kimberlin DW, Barnett ED, Lynfield R, et al. Red book: 2021–2024 report of the committee on infectious diseases. American Academy of Pediatrics; 2021.
2. Schillie S, Vellozzi C, Reingold A, et al. Prevention of hepatitis B virus infection in the United States: recommendations of the advisory committee on immunization practices. MMWR Recomm Rep (Morb Mortal Wkly Rep) 2018;67(1):1–31.
3. Hepatitis B virus: a comprehensive strategy for eliminating transmission in the United States through universal childhood vaccination. recommendations of the immunization practices advisory committee (ACIP). MMWR Recomm Rep (Morb Mortal Wkly Rep) 1991;40(Rr-13):1–25.
4. Coffin CS, Fung SK, Alvarez F, et al. Management of hepatitis B virus infection: 2018 guidelines from the canadian association for the study of liver disease and association of medical microbiology and infectious disease Canada. *Can Liver J.* 2018;1(4):156–217.
5. Global progress report on HIV, viral hepatitis and sexually transmitted infections, 2021. Accountability for the global health sector strategies 2016–2021: actions for impact. Geneva: World Health Organization; 2021.
6. Hepatitis B vaccine: Canadian Immunization Guide. Government of Canada. Available at: https://www.canada.ca/en/public-health/services/publications/healthy-living/canadian-immunization-guide-part-4-active-vaccines/page-7-hepatitis-b-vaccine.html#a51. Accessed November 8, 2022.
7. World Health Organization, Global health sector strategy on viral hepatitis 2016-2021. Towards ending viral hepatitis, Available at: https://apps.who.int/iris/handle/10665/246177, 2016. Accessed November 9, 2022.
8. Global health sector strategies on, respectively, HIV, viral hepatitis and sexually transmitted infections for the period 2022-2030. Geneva: World Health Organization; 2022.
9. U.S. Department of Health and Human Services, Viral hepatitis national strategic plan for the United States: a roadmap to elimination (2021-2025), Available at: https://www.hhs.gov/hepatitis/viral-hepatitis-national-strategic-plan/national-viral-hepatitis-action-plan-overview/index.html, 2020. Accessed November 9, 2022.
10. Din ES, Wasley A, Jacques-Carroll L, et al. Estimating the number of births to hepatitis B virus-infected women in 22 states, 2006. Pediatr Infect Dis J 2011;30(7):575–9.

11. Chung EK, Enquobahrie DA. Perinatal hepatitis B prevention: eliminating disease and disparity. Pediatrics 2021;147(3). https://doi.org/10.1542/peds.2020-037549.

12. Koneru A, Schillie S, Roberts H, et al. Estimating annual births to hepatitis B surface antigen–positive women in the united states by using data on maternal country of birth. Publ Health Rep 2019;134(3):255–63.

13. Cooke GS, Andrieux-Meyer I, Applegate TL, et al. Accelerating the elimination of viral hepatitis: a lancet gastroenterology & hepatology commission. *Lancet Gastroenterol Hepatol.* 2019;4(2):135–84.

14. Center for Disease Control and Prevention. Viral hepatitis surveillance - United States, 2019 2022. Available at: https://www.cdc.gov/hepatitis/statistics/2019surveillance/index.htm. Accessed September 29, 2022.

15. Roberts H, Ly KN, Yin S, et al. Prevalence of HBV infection, vaccine-induced immunity, and susceptibility among at-risk populations: US households, 2013-2018. Hepatology 2021;74(5):2353–65.

16. Wong RJ, Brosgart CL, Welch S, et al. An updated assessment of chronic hepatitis B prevalence among foreign-born persons living in the United States. Hepatology 2021;74(2):607–26.

17. Center for Disease Control and Prevention. Viral hepatitis surveillance - United States 2020. Available at: https://www.cdc.gov/hepatitis/statistics/2020surveillance/index.htm. Accessed November 3, 2022.

18. Koneru A, Fenlon N, Schillie S, et al. National perinatal hepatitis B prevention program: 2009–2017. Pediatrics 2021;147(3). https://doi.org/10.1542/peds.2020-1823.

19. Ko SC, Fan L, Smith EA, et al. Estimated annual perinatal hepatitis B virus infections in the United States, 2000-2009. *J Pediatric Infect Dis Soc.* 2016;5(2): 114–21.

20. Stevens CE, Toy PT, Tong MJ, et al. Perinatal hepatitis B virus transmission in the United States. prevention by passive-active immunization. JAMA 1985;253(12): 1740–5.

21. Chen HL, Lin LH, Hu FC, et al. Effects of maternal screening and universal immunization to prevent mother-to-infant transmission of HBV. Gastroenterology 2012; 142(4):773–81.e2.

22. Brown RS Jr, McMahon BJ, Lok AS, et al. Antiviral therapy in chronic hepatitis B viral infection during pregnancy: a systematic review and meta-analysis. Hepatology 2016;63(1):319–33.

23. Sookoian S. Liver disease during pregnancy: acute viral hepatitis. Ann Hepatol 2006;5(3):231–6.

24. Hill JB, Sheffield JS, Kim MJ, et al. Risk of hepatitis B transmission in breast-fed infants of chronic hepatitis B carriers. Obstet Gynecol 2002;99(6):1049–52.

25. Beasley RP, Stevens CE, Shiao IS, et al. Evidence against breast-feeding as a mechanism for vertical transmission of hepatitis B. Lancet 1975;2(7938):740–1.

26. Lewis E, Shinefield HR, Woodruff BA, et al. Safety of neonatal hepatitis B vaccine administration. Pediatr Infect Dis J 2001;20(11):1049–54.

27. Hepatitis B vaccination–United States, 1982-2002. MMWR Morb Mortal Wkly Rep 2002;51(25):549–52 , 563.

28. Commitee on Infectious Diseases Committee on Fetus Newborn. Elimination of Perinatal Hepatitis B: Providing the First Vaccine Dose Within 24 Hours of Birth. Pediatrics 2017;140(3). https://doi.org/10.1542/peds.2017-1870.

29. Khetsuriani N, Lesi O, Desai S, et al. Progress toward the elimination of mother-to-child transmission of hepatitis B virus - worldwide, 2016-2021. MMWR Morb Mortal Wkly Rep 2022;71(30):958–63.

30. Kolasa MS, Tsai Y, Xu J, et al. Hepatitis B surface antigen testing among pregnant women, United States 2014. Pediatr Infect Dis J 2017;36(7):e175–80.
31. Harris AM, Isenhour C, Schillie S, et al. Hepatitis B virus testing and care among pregnant women using commercial claims data, United States, 2011-2014. Infect Dis Obstet Gynecol 2018;2018:4107329.
32. Kubo A, Shlager L, Marks AR, et al. Prevention of vertical transmission of hepatitis B: an observational study. Ann Intern Med 2014;160(12):828–35.
33. Newborn hepatitis B vaccination coverage among children born January 2003-June 2005–United States. MMWR Morb Mortal Wkly Rep 2008;57(30):825 8.
34. Hill HA, Yankey D, Elam-Evans LD, et al. Vaccination coverage by age 24 months among children born in 2016 and 2017 - National Immunization Survey-Child, United States, 2017-2019. MMWR Morb Mortal Wkly Rep 2020;69(42):1505–11.
35. Pelts K, Lemma T. 2020 Hepatitis B birth dose and timely vaccination goals: Are we there yet? Pediatrics 2020;146(1_MeetingAbstract):554–6.
36. O'Leary ST, Nelson C, Duran J. Maternal characteristics and hospital policies as risk factors for nonreceipt of hepatitis B vaccine in the newborn nursery. Pediatr Infect Dis J 2012;31(1):1–4.
37. Willis BC, Wortley P, Wang SA, et al. Gaps in hospital policies and practices to prevent perinatal transmission of hepatitis B virus. Pediatrics 2010;125(4):704–11.
38. Dempsey AF, Schaffer S, Singer D, et al. Alternative vaccination schedule preferences among parents of young children. Pediatrics 2011;128(5):848–56.
39. Terrault NA, Lok ASF, McMahon BJ, et al. Update on prevention, diagnosis, and treatment of chronic hepatitis B: AASLD 2018 hepatitis B guidance. Hepatology 2018;67(4):1560–99.
40. American College of Obstetricians and Gynecologists' Immunization and Emerging Infections Expert Work Group. Hepatitis B prevention practice advisory 2021. Available at: https://www.acog.org/clinical/clinical-guidance/practice-advisory/articles/2018/01/hepatitis-b-prevention. Accessed September 29, 2022.
41. World Health Organization. Prevention of mother-to-child transmission of hepatitis B virus: guidelines on antiviral prophylaxis in pregnancy. Geneva: World Health Organization; 2020.
42. Dionne-Odom J, Tita AT, Silverman NS. 38: Hepatitis B in pregnancy screening, treatment, and prevention of vertical transmission. Am J Obstet Gynecol 2016;214(1):6–14.
43. Workowski KA, Bachmann LH, Chan PA, et al. Sexually transmitted infections treatment guidelines, 2021. MMWR Recomm Rep (Morb Mortal Wkly Rep) 2021;70(4):1–187.
44. Beasley RP, Hwang LY, Lee GC, et al. Prevention of perinatally transmitted hepatitis B virus infections with hepatitis B immune globulin and hepatitis B vaccine. Lancet 1983;2(8359):1099–102.
45. Nolt D, O'Leary ST, Aucott SW. Risks of infectious diseases in newborns exposed to alternative perinatal practices. Pediatrics 2022;149(2). https://doi.org/10.1542/peds.2021-055554. DISEASES COI, FETUS CO, NEWBORN.
46. Weng MK, Doshani M, Khan MA, et al. Universal hepatitis B vaccination in adults aged 19-59 years: updated recommendations of the advisory committee on immunization practices - United States, 2022. MMWR Morb Mortal Wkly Rep 2022;71(13):477–83.
47. Sirilert S, Tongsong T. Hepatitis B virus infection in pregnancy: an update on evidence-based management. Obstet Gynecol Surv 2020;75(9):557–65.

48. Nelson NP, Jamieson DJ, Murphy TV. Prevention of perinatal hepatitis B virus transmission. Journal of the Pediatric Infectious Diseases Society 2014; 3(suppl_1):S7–12.
49. Yang J, Zeng XM, Men YL, et al. Elective caesarean section versus vaginal delivery for preventing mother to child transmission of hepatitis B virus–a systematic review. Virol J 2008;5:100.
50. Meek JY, Noble L, Section on Breastfeeding. Policy statement: breastfeeding and the use of human milk. Pediatrics 2022;150(1). https://doi.org/10.1542/peds.2022-057988.
51. Immunizaton Action Coalition. Reducing medical errors: case reports. Available at: www.immunize.org/protect-newborns/guide/chapter2/case-reports.pdf. Accessed October 13, 2022.
52. Chao SD, Cheung CM, Chang ET, et al. Management of hepatitis B infected pregnant women: a cross-sectional study of obstetricians. BMC Pregnancy Childbirth 2019;19(1):275.

Hepatitis C Virus in Pregnancy
An Opportunity to Test and Treat

Rachel S. Fogel, BA[a], Catherine A. Chappell, MD, MSc[b,c,*]

KEYWORDS

- Hepatitis C • Pregnancy • Perinatal transmission • Direct-acting antivirals

KEY POINTS

- Injection drug use has led to a dramatic rise in the prevalence of hepatitis C virus (HCV) among pregnant people and, consequently, their infants.
- Linkage to care in the postpartum period for initiation of HCV treatment is the current standard of care, although studies have shown that greater than 90% of people do not receive treatment within the first year postpartum.
- Screening for infants with perinatal exposure is frequently missed, and utilization of HCV RNA testing as early as 2 months of age might improve infant screening rates.
- The use of direct-acting antivirals (DAAs) antenatally could both cure maternal HCV infection and prevent perinatal HCV transmission, but there are insufficient data on this strategy.
- Larger studies are needed to assess the safety and efficacy of DAA medications for use in pregnancy.

INTRODUCTION

An estimated 15 million people of childbearing potential have chronic hepatitis C virus (HCV) and are at risk for the development of cirrhosis and hepatocellular carcinoma.[1] Further, approximately 5% of pregnant people with HCV will vertically transmit HCV to their infants.[2] In the United States, injection drug use among people of reproductive age is the leading cause of new HCV infections and has resulted in a dramatic rise in the prevalence of HCV among pregnant people.[3] Pregnancy is a time of high health care engagement and a window of opportunity for HCV screening and linkage to HCV care. Utilization of direct-acting antivirals (DAAs) during pregnancy might not only cure maternal HCV but may also prevent perinatal HCV transmission.

[a] University of Pittsburgh School of Medicine, 3550 Terrace Street, Pittsburgh, PA 15213, USA; [b] Department of Obstetrics, Gynecology and Reproductive Sciences, Magee-Womens Hospital, 300 Halket Street, Pittsburgh, PA 15213, USA; [c] Magee-Womens Research Institute, 204 Craft Avenue, Pittsburgh, PA 15213, USA
* Corresponding author.
E-mail address: chappellca@upmc.edu

Obstet Gynecol Clin N Am 50 (2023) 363–373
https://doi.org/10.1016/j.ogc.2023.02.008

EPIDEMIOLOGY

HCV is a bloodborne pathogen that is transmitted via percutaneous exposure to blood from an infected person.[4] Sexual transmission of HCV is also possible and thought to be rare among heterosexual couples.[5] More recent data among men who have sex with men indicate that sexual transmission might be more common, especially with anal sex, high-risk sexual acts that could damage the mucosal barrier or cause bleeding, or with other sexually transmitted infections and/or concomitant drug use.[6] Though this article is not focused on men, these findings highlight that sexual transmission is possible and that certain sex practices might result in an increased risk of HCV acquisition.

Until the 2010s, HCV was thought of as a baby boomer disease, acquired primarily through health care exposures (through blood products and organ transplantation) or perinatal transmission in the 1940s to 1960s. However, the introduction of the abuse-deterrent formulation of OxyContin in 2010 in response to the worsening opioid epidemic in the United States led to the unintended consequence of a sharp increase in injection drug use. This rise corresponded with an increase in HCV infections among young people aged 20 to 39 years, leading to a dramatic shift in disease epidemiology such that this age group now accounts for the highest percentage of new cases of HCV.[7]

At the start of the COVID-19 pandemic in 2020, the United States saw a significant increase in opioid overdose deaths, up to 21.4 per 100,000 from 15.5 per 100,000 in 2019.[8,9] Simultaneously, the incidence of acute HCV infections rose from approximately 57,500 in 2019 to more than 66,700 in 2020. Among women of reproductive age (15–49 years), 21,909 cases of newly identified chronic HCV infection were reported in 2020, with 25 states reporting 165 cases of perinatal HCV infection that year.[7]

Between 2000 and 2015, the rate of HCV infection among pregnant people per 1000 live births in the United States increased from 0.8 to 4.1. Between 2011 and 2014 alone, an estimated 1700 infants were born with HCV infection.[10] Without adequate interventions to specifically target women of reproductive age with HCV, the prevalence of HCV will continue to increase, especially among persons of reproductive age and children.

PATHOGENESIS
Progression from Acute Infection to Cirrhosis and Hepatocellular Carcinoma

HCV is a spherical, enveloped, single-stranded RNA virus belonging to the family Flaviviridae. The single-stranded RNA codes for a single polyprotein that is then processed into 10 structural and regulatory proteins, and it replicates via an error-prone RNA-dependent RNA polymerase.[11,12] The virus primarily targets hepatocytes, but recent research has shown that HCV also infects B-lymphocytes, potentially improving immune evasion in the setting of chronic infection.[13]

Approximately 80% of acute infections are asymptomatic, whereas the other 20% may experience symptomatic hepatitis with symptoms including fever, malaise, loss of appetite, nausea, vomiting, dark urine, pale stool, and jaundice. The associated liver damage is due to the host immune response to the infected hepatocytes and can lead to fibrosis. Following initial exposure to the virus, roughly 15% to 25% of acute infections are cleared, while 75% to 85% become chronic. Only rarely do acute infections progress to fulminant hepatitis.[12–14] Young persons and women are more likely to spontaneously clear HCV.[15,16] Progression to cirrhosis occurs slowly, with 10% to 20% of people with chronic HCV developing cirrhosis over 20 years. Interestingly, progression to cirrhosis occurs more slowly in women, likely due to the antifibrotic effect of estrogen.[17] Once a person develops cirrhosis, however, the rate of progression to hepatocellular carcinoma is approximately 1% to 4% per year.[18]

Impact of Pregnancy on Hepatitis C Virus

There are few well-controlled studies of the impact of pregnancy on the course of HCV infection. Pregnancy appears to have minimal impact on HCV disease progression and indeed may even be beneficial for the long-term natural history of the disease due to increased estrogen exposure.[17,19] In addition, HCV RNA viral load increases during pregnancy whereas hepatocellular damage, and correspondingly, alanine aminotransferase, decrease, likely due to the relative immunosuppression seen in pregnancy.[20,21] However, in the immediate postpartum period, immune reconstitution occurs and can lead to a symptomatic flare, often with worsening hepatocellular damage.[22] Rarely, postpartum immune reconstitution may cause spontaneous HCV clearance.[23,24]

Impact of Hepatitis C Virus on Pregnancy

Like the impact of pregnancy on HCV, there are few well-controlled studies regarding the impact of HCV on both maternal and fetal pregnancy outcomes. Several studies have shown an increased likelihood of developing intrahepatic cholestasis of pregnancy (ICP) among those with active HCV infection (people with HCV viremia).[25–27] The pathophysiology behind this association remains unclear, although it has been postulated that the role of estrogen in cholestasis may be important.[26,28,29] In addition, some studies have suggested that people with active HCV infection may be more likely to develop gestational diabetes, though others have found no association or even the opposite effect.[27,30–32] Various studies have also shown increased rates of miscarriage, preterm birth, small for gestational age and low birthweight infants, need for a stay in the neonatal intensive care unit, and intrauterine fetal demise; however, it remains unclear whether these outcomes are due to infection with HCV or confounders such as continued intravenous drug use, alcohol consumption, or other social determinants of health.[33–35] For instance, one study investigating differences in obstetric outcomes for pregnant people with opioid use disorders (OUD) and HCV compared to pregnant people with OUD but not HCV found no difference in obstetric outcomes between groups but did find that people with OUD and HCV were more likely to have a history of incarceration, unstable housing, heroin use, other injection drug use, and overdose.[36]

Perinatal Transmission

Perinatal transmission of HCV represents the most common cause of HCV infection in infants and children. Studies have shown that 25% to 50% of HCV transmission events occur in early-to mid-pregnancy, 50% to 75% occur in late pregnancy, and 5% to 10% occur during delivery.[37–39] Limited data suggest that higher maternal HCV viral load, invasive fetal monitoring, prolonged rupture of membranes, and longer duration of labor may be associated with an increased likelihood of perinatal transmission.[40] Until recently, perinatal transmission of HCV to the fetus was believed to occur in approximately 5% of cases in the United States, with that rate doubling in the setting of human immunodeficiency virus (HIV) co-infection. Spontaneous clearance of HCV was thought to occur in 25% to 40% of cases by 5 years of age. However, a recent study estimates that the rate of perinatal transmission could be as high as 7.2% (12.1% with HCV/HIV co-infection) but with a rate of spontaneous clearance as high as 66% by age 5.[39,41]

Perinatal HCV infection is most often asymptomatic, and significant morbidity from HCV infection in children is uncommon.[42] Occasionally, children with HCV can have fatigue, abdominal pain, and/or hepatomegaly. Most children have mild aminotransferase elevations, yet severe liver fibrosis or cirrhosis is uncommon. Progression of HCV to cirrhosis and hepatocellular carcinoma rarely occurs before adulthood.[43]

DIAGNOSIS
Universal Screening in Pregnancy

Until recently, HCV screening during pregnancy was only conducted in individuals who were considered high risk.[44,45] However, this approach has been shown to be ineffective, as it relies on personal disclosure of often stigmatized behaviors, introduces physician bias, and frequently leads to missed diagnoses due to misjudgment of risk.[46–49] Thus, in 2018, the American Association for the Study of Liver Diseases (AASLD) and the Infectious Diseases Society of America (IDSA) jointly published updated guidance recommending that all persons who are pregnant be tested for HCV during each pregnancy, with the goal of identifying all cases of HCV so that pregnant people could be linked to care, and HCV-exposed infants could be screened. In March 2020, the United States Preventive Services Task Force (USPSTF) released an official recommendation that all people aged 18 to 79 years (including pregnant people) should be tested for HCV regardless of perceived risk factors.[44] The following month, the Centers for Disease Control and Prevention (CDC) followed suit, issuing a statement urging all prenatal care providers to test their pregnant patients during each pregnancy due to the rising rate of HCV infection among young adults aged 20 to 39.[50] Finally, in May 2021, the American College of Obstetricians and Gynecologists (ACOG) published a practice bulletin citing both the USPSTF and CDC recommendations and officially recommending that HCV testing be performed at all initial prenatal visits.[51] In accordance with the recommendations put forth by AASLD/IDSA, the USPSTF, the CDC, and ACOG, a testing algorithm for HCV screening should be implemented during the initial prenatal visit for all pregnant persons (**Fig. 1**). HCV screening should be conducted using reflex testing, meaning that any sample found to be HCV IgG seropositive should automatically have an HCV RNA test. This is an efficient strategy that can determine the HCV status of a person with only one blood draw. Consideration should also be made for repeat HCV testing in the third trimester or at delivery for those who continue to have a high-risk exposure, such as ongoing injection drug use.

MANAGEMENT OF HEPATITIS C VIRUS INFECTION
Antepartum

Although the USPSTF, CDC, AASLD/IDSA, and ACOG screening guidelines recommend testing for HCV at the initial prenatal visit, there are currently no interventions available to impact maternal HCV infection or to prevent perinatal transmission of HCV. The primary goal during the antepartum period should be to connect the pregnant person with an HCV treatment provider. Unfortunately, several studies have shown that few people who test positive for HCV during their pregnancies actually receive treatment at any point in the postpartum period.[52,53] One large retrospective cohort study exploring the prevalence of HCV testing in pregnancy and postpartum follow-up for treatment among people with OUD found that of the 19,697 people who were followed for 6 months postpartum, fewer than 6% attended a follow-up visit or received treatment during that time.[54] This highlights the logistical challenges that are faced during the postpartum period and that linkage during antenatal care might

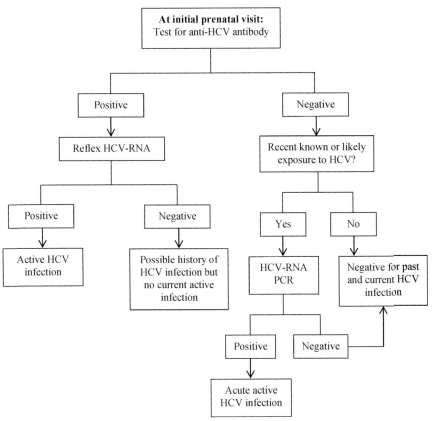

Fig. 1. Testing algorithm for initial prenatal visit (or first prenatal visit during which labs are drawn) to screen for active HCV infection.

be more successful. In the last decade, HCV treatment has been revolutionized such that now treatment is orally administered for 8 to 12 weeks and is well-tolerated, with a greater than 95% cure rate. With the advent of DAAs, everyone should know their HCV status so they can be cured, and treatment should be easily accessible. Providers treating HCV postpartum should focus on reducing barriers to treatment, such as using a simplified strategy for treatment, utilizing telemedicine, and delivering HCV treatment to the patient's home.[55]

Additionally, providers should discuss reducing other potential hepatoxic agents, such as limiting acetaminophen use to 2 g or less per day, as well as quitting smoking. Hepatitis A and B vaccination should be given if the patient is non-immune during pregnancy.[54] Providers should also educate their patients about the symptoms of ICP and should maintain a low threshold to test for elevated bile acids given the increased risk in the context of active HCV infection.[25–27] Additionally, while no studies to date have shown that invasive prenatal testing (eg, amniocentesis, chorionic villous sampling) leads to increased rates of perinatal transmission of HCV, the Society for Maternal-Fetal Medicine (SMFM) has recommended that providers counsel their patients that available data regarding risk of perinatal transmission are encouraging but limited.[56,57]

Intrapartum

Several studies have suggested that some intrapartum interventions, including internal fetal monitoring (ie, with a fetal scalp electrode), operative delivery, and episiotomy, may increase the likelihood of perinatal transmission at the time of delivery.[40,58,59] SMFM thus recommends avoiding these interventions unless necessary in the course of management.[57] However, while this guidance is theoretically helpful, in practice, these interventions are not typically utilized unless in situations where the provider deems it to be medically necessary for the health and safety of the pregnant person or the neonate. In addition, two cohort studies found that prolonged rupture of membranes (>6 hours) increases the risk of transmission.[40,59] Early artificial rupture of membranes should therefore be avoided.[57]

There is currently no evidence to suggest that the mode of delivery impacts the rate of perinatal transmission, and therefore, elective cesarean delivery is not recommended solely for the purpose of lowering HCV transmission risk.[19,37,60–63] However, these studies may have been underpowered. Furthermore, most studies investigating this association did not differentiate between elective and emergent cesarean sections and are thus difficult to interpret given the difference in risk factors (eg, higher risk of transmission with contractions vs without).

Postpartum

The primary goals of management in the postpartum period include linkage to care with an infectious diseases or hepatology provider, as well as documentation of the need for future testing for the infant. A meta-analysis including 14 studies examining the risk of HCV transmission via breast- or chest-feeding found no associations between avoidance of breast- or chest-feeding and reduced transmission rates.[64] Providers should therefore encourage their patients to breast- or chest-feed their infants unless they have cracked or bleeding nipples.[57]

Cross-placental transfer of anti-HCV IgG can persist in infant circulation for up to 18 months postpartum and therefore may not reliably be tested immediately. In addition, while transmission may occur in up to 6% to 8% of cases, many of these infections are spontaneously cleared by the age of 5.[39] Thus, it is not useful to rely on testing done immediately after birth. The AASLD and IDSA recommend testing for HCV RNA at >2 months or anti-HCV antibodies at 18 months. However, less than one-third of children who are exposed to HCV perinatally are screened when utilizing HCV antibody testing at 18 months. This may be due to children having changed pediatricians by 18 months or having been lost from primary pediatric care, or their birth exposures may have been forgotten.[47,65] Screening infants earlier with HCV RNA testing could improve screening rates among children who have been perinatally exposed to HCV. If the child is found to have HCV, they should then be re-tested for HCV RNA at 3 years to evaluate for spontaneous clearance.[66] If, at 3 years, the child is persistently positive, the provider should proceed with treatment, as DAAs have been approved for use in children 3 years or older.[45,66,67]

CURRENT STUDIES OF HEPATITIS C VIRUS TREATMENT IN PREGNANCY

The ideal model of care for pregnant people is universal HCV testing and treatment integrated into prenatal care, a time of high engagement and unique motivation. These gaps could be addressed by the utilization of DAAs for antenatal HCV treatment, which could cure maternal HCV infection as well as prevent HCV transmission. An encouraging phase 1 trial investigating the pharmacokinetics, safety, and efficacy of ledipasvir-sofosbuvir in nine pregnant people found no safety concerns and achieved a 100% cure rate with no cases of perinatal transmission.[67] However, this study also found that 34% of pregnant people screened were ineligible for participation because they had genotype 2 or 3 infection; therefore, a pan-genotypic treatment regimen would be more optimal. A pharmacokinetic study of sofosbuvir/velpatasvir HCV treatment in pregnant people (ClinicalTrials.gov Identifier: NCT04382404) recently completed enrollment, and a multicenter safety study of this same regimen in approximately 100 pregnant people (ClinicalTrials.gov Identifier: NCT05140941) is actively recruiting. The data from these clinical trials and an observational study of mother–infant outcomes following antenatal exposure to DAAs called the "Treatment in Pregnancy for Hepatitis C ("TiP-HepC") Registry" will provide additional supportive safety data (https://www.globalhep.org/evidence-base/treatment-pregnancy-hepatitis-c-tip-hepc-registry). DAAs have revolutionized treatment of HCV such that disease eradication is now within reach. It is clear, however, that without the ability to treat HCV during pregnancy, eradication will be IMPOSSIBLE.[68]

SUMMARY

One significant consequence of the opioid epidemic is the rise of HCV infection among persons of reproductive age, including pregnant people. Though there are adverse obstetric and neonatal outcomes associated with HCV, such as preterm birth and fetal growth restriction, it is difficult to determine whether these outcomes are due directly to HCV or other confounders such as substance use or social determinants of health. One significant outcome is that HCV can be perinatally transmitted, and currently, there are no interventions available to prevent transmission. DAAs have revolutionized HCV treatment, as they are orally administered, well-tolerated, and highly effective and are becoming increasingly accessible utilizing a simplified treatment strategy. Ideally, HCV treatment would occur before pregnancy; however, there is not currently an effective HCV screening and treatment pathway for reproductive-aged persons. Pregnant persons often learn they have HCV now that universal screening of HCV in pregnancy is recommended. Unfortunately, postpartum treatment currently has poor engagement, and thus, it is challenging to treat HCV before the next pregnancy. HCV treatment during pregnancy could be an ideal window of opportunity, as pregnancy is a time of high health care engagement, and pregnant persons might be uniquely motivated if antenatal treatment is shown to prevent perinatal HCV transmission. Studies are ongoing to evaluate the safety and efficacy of HCV DAA treatment during pregnancy.

CLINICS CARE POINTS

- Universal HCV screening utilizing reflex testing should be implemented for all pregnant people at the initial prenatal visit and should be repeated during the third trimester or at delivery if the patient continues to have high-risk exposures.

- Infants who are perinatally exposed to HCV are inadequately screened, and utilization of HCV RNA tests as early as 2 months of age could improve the screening rate.

- Simplified postpartum treatment utilizing telemedicine reduces barriers to care and may more effectively engage people who would otherwise be lost to follow-up.

- Treatment of HCV during pregnancy is currently undergoing evaluation and could result in curative maternal treatment and prevention of perinatal transmission of HCV.

DISCLOSURE

R.S. Fogel has nothing to disclose. C.A. Chappell has received research funding and consultation fees from Gilead Sciences and has received research grants from Merck and Organon.

REFERENCES

1. Dugan E, Blach S, Biondi M, et al. Global prevalence of hepatitis C virus in women of childbearing age in 2019: a modelling study. Lancet Gastroenterol Hepatol 2021;6(3). https://doi.org/10.1016/S2468-1253(20)30359-9.
2. Benova L, Mohamoud YA, Calvert C, et al. Vertical transmission of hepatitis C virus: systematic review and meta-analysis. Clin Infect Dis 2014;59(6):765–73.
3. Schillie SF, Canary L, Koneru A, et al. Hepatitis C virus in women of childbearing age, pregnant women, and children. Am J Prev Med 2018;55(5):633–41.
4. Thursz M, Fontanet A. HCV transmission in industrialized countries and resource-constrained areas. Nat Rev Gastroenterol Hepatol 2014;11(1):28–35.
5. Terrault NA, Dodge JL, Murphy EL, et al. Sexual transmission of hepatitis C virus among monogamous heterosexual couples: The HCV partners study. Hepatology 2013;57(3):881–9.
6. Nijmeijer BM, Koopsen J, Schinkel J, et al. Sexually transmitted hepatitis C virus infections: current trends, and recent advances in understanding the spread in men who have sex with men. J Int AIDS Soc 2019;22(S6). https://doi.org/10.1002/jia2.25348.
7. Hepatitis C Surveillance 2020. Centers for Disease Control and Prevention. 2020. Available at: https://www.cdc.gov/hepatitis/statistics/2020surveillance/hepatitis-c.htm. Accessed November 2, 2022.
8. Overdose Death Rates Involving Opioids, by Type, United States, 1999-2020. Centers for Disease Control and Prevention. 2022. Available at: https://www.cdc.gov/drugoverdose/data/od-death-data.html. Accessed November 2, 2022.
9. Ghose R, Forati AM, Mantsch JR. Impact of the COVID-19 pandemic on opioid overdose deaths: a spatiotemporal analysis. J Urban Health 2022;99(2):316–27.
10. HCV Infection. Centers for Disease Control and Prevention. 2022. Available at: https://www.cdc.gov/nchhstp/pregnancy/effects/hcv.html. Accessed November 2, 2022.
11. Dubuisson J. Hepatitis C virus proteins. World J Gastroenterol 2007;13(17):2406.
12. World Health Organization. Background - Epidemiology and Natural History. In: WHO Guidelines on Hepatitis B and C Testing. 2017. Available at: https://www.ncbi.nlm.nih.gov/books/NBK442290/. Accessed November 2, 2022.
13. Desombere I, van Houtte F, Farhoudi A, et al. A role for b cells to transmit hepatitis C Virus infection. Front Immunol 2021;12. https://doi.org/10.3389/fimmu.2021.775098.
14. Axley P, Ahmed Z, Ravi S, et al. Hepatitis C virus and hepatocellular carcinoma: a narrative review. J Clin Transl Hepatol 2018;6(2):1–6.
15. Rolfe KJ, Curran MD, Alexander GJM, et al. Spontaneous loss of hepatitis C virus RNA from serum is associated with genotype 1 and younger age at exposure. J Med Virol 2011;83(8):1338–44.
16. Fedorchenko Sv, Klimenko A, Martynovich T, et al. IL-28B genetic variation, gender, age, jaundice, hepatitis C virus genotype, and hepatitis B virus and HIV co-infection in spontaneous clearance of hepatitis C virus. Turk J Gastroenterol 2019;30(5):436–44.

17. di Martino V, Lebray P, Myers RP, et al. Progression of liver fibrosis in women infected with hepatitis C: Long-term benefit of estrogen exposure. Hepatology 2004;40(6):1426–33.
18. Chen SL, Morgan TR. The Natural History of Hepatitis C Virus (HCV) Infection. Int J Med Sci 2006;47–52. https://doi.org/10.7150/ijms.3.47.
19. Kushner T, Terrault NA. Hepatitis C in pregnancy: a unique opportunity to improve the hepatitis C cascade of care. Hepatol Commun 2019;3(1):20–8.
20. Irshad M, Gupta P, Irshad K. Immunopathogenesis of liver injury during hepatitis C virus infection. Viral Immunol 2019;32(3):112–20.
21. Gervais A, Bacq Y, Bernuau J, et al. Decrease in serum ALT and increase in serum HCV RNA during pregnancy in women with chronic hepatitis C. J Hepatol 2000;32(2):293–9.
22. Singh N, Perfect JR. Immune reconstitution syndrome and exacerbation of infections after pregnancy. Clin Infect Dis 2007;45(9):1192–9.
23. Hashem M, Jhaveri R, Saleh DA, et al. Spontaneous viral load decline and subsequent clearance of chronic hepatitis c virus in postpartum women correlates with favorable interleukin-28B gene allele. Clin Infect Dis 2017;65(6):999–1005.
24. Hattori Y, Orito E, Ohno T, et al. Loss of hepatitis C virus RNA after parturition in female patients with chronic HCV infection. J Med Virol 2003;71(2):205–11.
25. Paternoster DM, Fabris F, Palù G, et al. Intra-hepatic cholestasis of pregnancy in hepatitis C virus infection. Acta Obstet Gynecol Scand 2002;81(2):99–103.
26. Floreani A, Gervasi MT. New Insights on Intrahepatic Cholestasis of Pregnancy. Clin Liver Dis 2016;20(1):177–89.
27. Kushner T, Djerboua M, Biondi MJ, et al. Influence of hepatitis C viral parameters on pregnancy complications and risk of mother-to-child transmission. J Hepatol 2022;77(5):1256–64.
28. Chen J, Zhao K nan, Liu G bin. Estrogen-induced cholestasis: pathogenesis and therapeutic implications. Hepato-Gastroenterology 2013;60(126):1289–96.
29. Bacq Y, Sentilhes L. Intrahepatic cholestasis of pregnancy: diagnosis and management. Clin Liver Dis 2014;4(3):58–61.
30. Pergam SA, Wang CC, Gardella CM, et al. Pregnancy complications associated with hepatitis C: data from a 2003-2005 Washington state birth cohort. Am J Obstet Gynecol 2008;199(1):38.e1–9.
31. Connell LE, Salihu HM, Salemi JL, et al. Maternal hepatitis B and hepatitis C carrier status and perinatal outcomes. Liver Int 2011;31(8):1163–70.
32. Buresi MC, Lee J, Gill S, et al. The prevalence of gestational diabetes mellitus and glucose abnormalities in pregnant women with hepatitis C virus infection in british columbia. J Obstet Gynaecol Can 2010;32(10):935–41.
33. Karampatou A, Han X, Kondili LA, et al. Premature ovarian senescence and a high miscarriage rate impair fertility in women with HCV. J Hepatol 2018;68(1):33–41.
34. Money D, Boucoiran I, Wagner E, et al. Obstetrical and neonatal outcomes among women infected with hepatitis C and their infants. J Obstet Gynaecol Can 2014;36(9):785–94.
35. Chen B, Wang Y, Lange M, et al. Hepatitis C is associated with more adverse pregnancy outcomes than hepatitis B: a 7-year national inpatient sample study. Hepatol Commun 2022. https://doi.org/10.1002/hep4.2002.
36. Beermann SE, Porcelli BA, Durkin MJ, et al. The impact of hepatitis C on obstetric outcomes in an opioid use disorder-specific prenatal clinic. Am J Obstet Gynecol 2022;226(1):S378–9.

37. Resti M, Azzari C, Mannelli F, et al. Mother to child transmission of hepatitis C virus: prospective study of risk factors and timing of infection in children born to women seronegative for HIV-1. BMJ 1998;317(7156):437–41.

38. le Campion A, Larouche A, Fauteux-Daniel S, et al. Pathogenesis of hepatitis C during pregnancy and childhood. Viruses 2012;4(12). https://doi.org/10.3390/v4123531.

39. Ades AE, Gordon F, Scott K, et al. Overall vertical transmission of hepatitis C virus, transmission net of clearance, and timing of transmission. Clin Infect Dis 2022. https://doi.org/10.1093/cid/ciac270.

40. Mast EE, Hwang L, Seto DSY, et al. Risk factors for perinatal transmission of hepatitis C Virus (HCV) and the natural history of HCV infection acquired in infancy. J Infect Dis 2005;192(11):1880–9.

41. Ades AE, Gordon F, Scott K, et al. Spontaneous clearance of vertically acquired hepatitis c infection: implications for testing and treatment. Clin Infect Dis 2022. https://doi.org/10.1093/cid/ciac255.

42. Squires RH, Shneider BL, Bucuvalas J, et al. Acute liver failure in children: the first 348 patients in the pediatric acute liver failure study group. J Pediatr 2006;148(5):652–8.e2.

43. Leung DH, Squires JE, Jhaveri R, et al. Hepatitis C in 2020: a north american society for pediatric gastroenterology, hepatology, and nutrition position paper. J Pediatr Gastroenterol Nutr 2020;71(3):407–17.

44. Owens DK, Davidson KW, Krist AH, et al. Screening for hepatitis C VIRUS INFECTION IN ADOLESCENTS AND Adults. JAMA 2020;323(10):970.

45. Smith BD, Morgan RL, Beckett GA, et al. Recommendations for the identification of chronic hepatitis C virus infection among persons born during 1945-1965. MMWR Recomm Rep (Morb Mortal Wkly Rep) 2012;61(RR-4):1–32.

46. Kuncio DE, Newbern EC, Fernandez-Viña MH, et al. Comparison of risk-based hepatitis C screening and the true seroprevalence in an urban prison system. J Urban Health 2015;92(2):379–86.

47. Kuncio DE, Newbern EC, Johnson CC, et al. Failure to test and identify perinatally infected children born to hepatitis C virus–infected women. Clin Infect Dis 2016;62(8):980–5.

48. Waruingi W, Mhanna MJ, Kumar D, et al. Hepatitis C Virus universal screening versus risk based selective screening during pregnancy. J Neonatal Perinatal Med 2016;8(4):371–8.

49. Boudova S, Mark K, El-Kamary SS. Risk-based hepatitis C screening in pregnancy is less reliable than universal screening: a retrospective chart review. Open Forum Infect Dis 2018;5(3).

50. Test for Hepatitis C During Every Pregnancy. Centers for Disease Control and Prevention. 2021. Available at: https://www.cdc.gov/knowmorehepatitis/hcp/test-for-hepc-during-pregnancy.htm. Accessed November 2, 2022.

51. Hughes B, Jamieson DJ, Kaimal AJ, Caughey AB, Eke A, McReynolds M. Routine Hepatitis C Virus Screening in Pregnant Individuals. In: ACOG Practice Advisory. 2021. Available at: https://www.acog.org/clinical/clinical-guidance/practice-advisory/articles/2021/05/routine-hepatitis-c-virus-screening-in-pregnant-individuals. Accessed November 3, 2022.

52. Krans EE, Zickmund SL, Rustgi VK, et al. Screening and evaluation of hepatitis C virus infection in pregnant women on opioid maintenance therapy: a retrospective cohort study. Subst Abus 2016;37(1):88–95.

53. Bushman ET, Subramani L, Sanjanwala A, et al. Pragmatic experience with risk-based versus universal hepatitis C screening in pregnancy: detection of infection

and postpartum linkage to care. Am J Perinatol 2021;38(11). https://doi.org/10.1055/s-0041-1728827.

54. Jarlenski M, Chen Q, Ahrens KA, et al. Postpartum follow-up care for pregnant persons with opioid use disorder and hepatitis C virus infection. Obstet Gynecol 2022;139(5):916–8.

55. American Association for the Study of Liver Diseases, Infectious Diseases Society of America. Simplified HCV Treatment for Treatment-Naive Adults Without Cirrhosis. In: HCV Guidance: Recommendations for Testing, Managing, and Treating Hepatitis C. 2022. Available at: https://www.hcvguidelines.org/treatment-naive/simplified-treatment. Accessed November 3, 2022.

56. Wilson RD. Guideline No. 409: intrauterine fetal diagnostic testing in women with chronic viral infections. J Obstet Gynaecol Can 2020;42(12):1555–62.e1.

57. Dotters-Katz SK, Kuller JA, Hughes BL. Society for maternal-fetal medicine consult series #56: hepatitis c in pregnancy—updated guidelines. Am J Obstet Gynecol 2021;225(3):B8–18.

58. Garcia-Tejedor A, Maiques-Montesinos V, Diago-Almela VJ, et al. Risk factors for vertical transmission of hepatitis C virus: a single center experience with 710 HCV-infected mothers. Eur J Obstet Gynecol Reprod Biol 2015;194:173–7.

59. Spencer JD, Latt N, Beeby PJ, et al. Transmission of hepatitis C virus to infants of human immunodeficiency virus-negative intravenous drug-using mothers: rate of infection and assessment of risk factors for transmission. J Viral Hepat 1997;4(6):395–409.

60. Pembrey L, Pier-Angelo T, Newell ML. Effects of mode of delivery and infant feeding on the risk of mother-to-child transmission of hepatitis C virus. BJOG 2001;108(4):371–7.

61. European Paediatric Hepatitis C Virus Network. A significant sex—but not elective cesarean section—effect on mother-to-child transmission of hepatitis C virus infection. J Infect Dis 2005;192(11):1872–9.

62. McMenamin MB, Jackson AD, Lambert J, et al. Obstetric management of hepatitis C-positive mothers: analysis of vertical transmission in 559 mother-infant pairs. Am J Obstet Gynecol 2008;199(3):315.e1–5.

63. Ghamar Chehreh ME, Tabatabaei SV, Khazanehdari S, et al. Effect of cesarean section on the risk of perinatal transmission of hepatitis C virus from HCV-RNA+/HIV− mothers: a meta-analysis. Arch Gynecol Obstet 2011;283(2):255–60.

64. Cottrell EB, Chou R, Wasson N, et al. Reducing risk for mother-to-infant transmission of hepatitis C virus: a systematic review for the U.S. preventive services task force. Ann Intern Med 2013;158(2):109.

65. Chappell CA, Hillier SL, Crowe D, et al. Hepatitis C virus screening among children exposed during pregnancy. Pediatrics 2018;141(6). https://doi.org/10.1542/peds.2017-3273.

66. American Association for the Study of Liver Diseases, Infectious Diseases Society of America. HCV in Children. In: HCV Guidance: Recommendations for Testing, Managing, and Treating Hepatitis C. 2022. Available at: https://www.hcvguidelines.org/unique-populations/children. Accessed November 3, 2022.

67. Chappell CA, Scarsi KK, Kirby BJ, et al. Ledipasvir plus sofosbuvir in pregnant women with hepatitis C virus infection: a phase 1 pharmacokinetic study. Lancet Microbe 2020;1(5):e200–8.

68. Jhaveri R, Yee LM, Antala S, et al. Responsible inclusion of pregnant individuals in eradicating HCV. Hepatology 2021;74(3). https://doi.org/10.1002/hep.31825.

Group B Streptococcus in Pregnancy

Jenny Y. Mei, MD, Neil S. Silverman, MD*

KEYWORDS

- Group B streptococcus • Neonatal sepsis • Intrapartum antibiotic prophylaxis

KEY POINTS

- All pregnant patients should undergo antepartum Group B streptococcus (GBS) screening between 36 0/7 and 37 6/7 weeks of gestation, regardless of planned mode of birth.
- Patients with GBS bacteriuria, a history of newborn with GBS disease, or positive GBS vaginal-rectal culture at any point in the pregnancy should receive intrapartum antibiotic prophylaxis (IAP), with the exception of those undergoing a prelabor cesarean delivery with intact membranes.
- If GBS status is unknown at the time of labor onset, IAP should be administered in the setting of the following risk factors for GBS early-onset disease: risk of preterm birth, preterm prelabor rupture of membranes, rupture of membranes for 18 or more hours at term, or intrapartum fever (temperature 100.4°F [38°C] or higher).
- The antibiotic of choice for GBS prophylaxis is intravenous penicillin; cefazolin is the recommended alternative for patients with low-risk penicillin allergies.
- Patients with high-risk penicillin allergies should have their GBS isolate evaluated for clindamycin susceptibility; otherwise, vancomycin should be administered.

INTRODUCTION

Group B streptococcus (GBS) is the leading cause of newborn infection, with the primary risk factor being maternal colonization of the genitourinary and gastrointestinal tracts.[1] Maternal-fetal/neonatal transmission most commonly occurs during labor.[2] Implementation of universal intrapartum antibiotic prophylaxis (IAP) has reduced the incidence of GBS early-onset disease (GBS EOD) from 1.8 newborns per 1000 live births in the 1990s to 0.23 newborns per 1000 live births in 2015.[3]

Specific prenatal interventions have been identified as key to decreasing the risk for GBS EOD:[4]

- Universal prenatal screening for maternal vaginal-rectal GBS colonization
- Proper GBS test specimen collection and processing

Division of Maternal-Fetal Medicine, Department of Obstetrics and Gynecology, David Geffen School of Medicine at UCLA, 200 Medical Plaza, Suite 430, Los Angeles, CA 90095-1740, USA
* Corresponding author.
E-mail address: NSSilverman@mednet.ucla.edu

Obstet Gynecol Clin N Am 50 (2023) 375–387
https://doi.org/10.1016/j.ogc.2023.02.009
0889-8545/23/© 2023 Elsevier Inc. All rights reserved.

obgyn.theclinics.com

- Appropriate implementation of IAP in colonized pregnant patients
- Coordination with pediatric care providers for targeted surveillance of at-risk newborns

Although these measures cannot eliminate all cases, implementation of these strategies will significantly reduce the incidence of GBS EOD and its associated morbidities.

CLINICAL RELEVANCE

GBS emerged in the 1970s as a major cause of perinatal morbidity and mortality in newborns.[2,5,6] There are two clinical syndromes of invasive GBS disease in the newborn: GBS EOD and GBS late-onset disease.

GBS EOD occurs due to vertical transmission or fetal/neonatal aspiration during labor and delivery. It presents within 7 days of birth, most commonly within 12 to 48 h, as sepsis, pneumonia, or meningitis.[1,7,8] Overall, GBS EOD is the most common cause of early-onset neonatal sepsis and the main focus of prevention through IAP.[9]

On the contrary, GBS late-onset disease is acquired via horizontal transmission from the mother after birth, or during the infant's hospital stay, or in their household.[10] It presents between 7 days and 3 months of age as bacteremia or meningitis, with other systemic symptoms also reported.[10]

It is estimated that 50% of infants born to GBS-colonized mothers will be colonized with GBS, with 1% to 2% of colonized term newborns developing GBS EOD in the absence of IAP during labor.[5,11] Although the majority (72%) of GBS EOD cases occur in term newborns, morbidity and mortality are significantly higher in preterm newborns (19.2%) compared with those delivered at term (2.1%).[3,12]

PRENATAL RISKS

GBS is a facultative gram-positive organism physiologically present in the intestinal and vaginal microbiome of some patients; the gastrointestinal tract serves as the primary reservoir for the bacteria. Prevalence of colonization among pregnant patients ranges between 10% to 30% and may be intermittent, transitory, or persistent.[13,14]

Although largely asymptomatic in the nonpregnant patient, GBS colonization can cause maternal urinary tract infections and intraamniotic infection, as well as postpartum endometritis.[7,15,16] It has also been associated with preterm labor and stillbirth. Specifically, when maternal colonization was identified through a diagnosis of GBS bacteriuria, which has been shown to be related to higher levels of genitourinary colonization overall, the association with preterm birth was found to be significantly higher (relative risk [RR] 1.98; 95% confidence interval [CI], 1.45 to 2.69; $P < .001$).[17]

GENERAL GUIDELINES

Maternal vaginal-rectal colonization with GBS is the main risk factor for neonatal GBS EOD.[6] Other risk factors associated with GBS EOD include prematurity, very low birth weight, prolonged rupture of membranes, intraamniotic infection, and young maternal age.[3,17] There have also been increased risks for GBS EOD associated with heavy colonization, GBS bacteriuria, and having a previous newborn affected by GBS EOD.[18,19] GBS detected in a urine specimen at any colony count serves as a marker for heavy colonization, even if the bacterial level is below the cutoff recommended for asymptomatic treatment [10^5 colony-forming units (CFU)/mL].

Intravenous IAP is recommended to prevent GBS EOD in infants born to women with positive GBS cultures or who have other risk factors for intrapartum colonization.[11]

Alternative methods have not been shown to be comparably effective and are not recommended, including the use of oral or intramuscular antibiotic regimens before or during labor, as well as substituting antibiotics with vaginal antiseptics.[20,21]

The most recent guidelines from the American College of Obstetrics and Gynecologists (ACOG) now recommend antepartum GBS screening at 36 0/7 to 37 6/7 weeks of gestation regardless of planned mode of birth.[4] Patients who have GBS bacteriuria during pregnancy or a history of a GBS EOD-affected newborn do not need antepartum GBS screening and should receive IAP outright.

Group B Streptococcus Screening: Timing and Methods

The predictive ability of GBS screening results, both by culture and polymerase chain reaction techniques, has been shown to significantly after 5 weeks from sample collection.[22,23] The revised timing for antepartum screening (36 0/7 to 37 6/7 weeks) now provides a 5-week window for valid culture results up to a gestational age of 41 0/7 weeks.

Proper GBS test collection employs a single swab to obtain a sample first from the lower vagina (near the introitus), then the rectum (through the anal sphincter).[4] This method of sampling is important, as it significantly increases test yield as compared with sampling the cervix or vagina alone.[22,24] For patients who wish to collect their own samples, similar yields, after focused education, to health provider collection have been shown.[25]

Molecular-Based Nucleic-Acid Testing for Group B Streptococcus

Nucleic-acid amplification testing (NAAT) for GBS has been shown to be equivalent to or even more sensitive than culture-based screening for GBS detection, but only when a similar incubation step for the sample in enrichment broth is used before final laboratory analysis.[26,27]

Of note, in contrast to culture, NAAT does not isolate the organism, so cannot allow for antibiotic susceptibility testing of a GBS-positive sample. Therefore, laboratories should be made aware when specimens are from patients with high-risk penicillin (PCN) allergies, so that a corollary culture-based screening with appropriate susceptibility testing can also be performed.

NAAT point-of-care testing has been considered as a rapid test for patients who present in labor with unknown or unavailable GBS test results, due to its potential ability to provide results before the patient delivers. However, without an enrichment broth incubation step, sensitivity rates for this use of an NAAT GBS test are lower, with up to 7% to 10% failure rates reported.[27] If GBS testing by NAAT is used in this manner, a positive test can be used to start IAP, but a negative test result should default to the use of risk factors as a guide for starting antibiotics, until such time that negative predictive values for unincubated NAATs for GBS can be technically reduced.[4]

INDICATIONS FOR INTRAPARTUM ANTIBIOTIC PROPHYLAXIS

The standard, most common indications for starting IAP for GBS are outlined in **Table 1**. Other potential scenarios include.

- Patients with a positive GBS test result who undergo a cesarean delivery before the onset of labor and with intact membranes do not require IAP[28]
- Patients who have a positive GBS test result at any point in pregnancy, including those with resolved preterm labor without delivery, do not need to have repeat testing later in pregnancy and should be treated with IAP[29]
- If GBS status is unknown at the onset of labor, IAP should be administered according to the established risk factors for GBS EOD

Table 1
Intrapartum antibiotic prophylaxis for prevention of neonatal group B streptococcus early-onset disease

Intrapartum GBS Prophylaxis Indicated	Intrapartum GBS Prophylaxis Not Indicated
Maternal History	
Previous neonate with invasive GBS disease	GBS colonization during a previous pregnancy[a]
Current Pregnancy	
Positive GBS culture obtained at 36 0/7 wk of gestation or more during the current pregnancy[b]	Negative GBS culture obtained at 36 0/7 wk of gestation or more during the current pregnancy
Positive GBS culture obtained at any point previously in the pregnancy and anticipate delivery[c]	Negative GBS culture obtained in the past 5 wk and anticipate delivery
GBS bacteriuria anytime in the current pregnancy	Cesarean birth performed before onset of labor with intact amniotic membranes (regardless of GBS colonization status or gestational age)
Intrapartum	
Unknown GBS status at onset of labor with any of the following risk factors below:	Negative GBS culture obtained at 36 0/7 wk of gestation or more during the current pregnancy, regardless of intrapartum risk factors
Anticipated birth <37 0/7 wk of gestation	Negative GBS culture obtained in the last 5 wk, regardless of intrapartum risk factors
Amniotic membrane rupture 18 h or greater	Unknown GBS status with no intrapartum risk factors[e]
Intrapartum temperature 100.4°F (38°C) or higher[d]	
Intrapartum NAAT result positive for GBS	
Intrapartum NAAT results negative but risk factors develop	
Known GBS-positive status in a previous pregnancy	

Abbreviations: GBS, group B streptococcus; NAAT, nucleic acid amplification test.
   [a] Unless GBS status in current pregnancy is unknown at onset of labor at term.
   [b] Unless cesarean birth is performed before the onset of labor with intact amniotic membranes.
   [c] Patients with positive GBS culture at any point in pregnancy do not need repeat testing and should be treated with intrapartum antibiotic prophylaxis.
   [d] If intraamniotic infection is suspected, broad-spectrum antibiotic therapy should replace GBS prophylaxis, including an agent that treats GBS.
   [e] Risk factors include gestational age less than 37 0/7 wk, amniotic membrane rupture 18 h or greater, maternal temperature 100.4°F (38°C) or higher.
   Verani JR, McGee L, Schrag SJ. Prevention of perinatal group B streptococcal disease—revised guidelines from CDC, 2010. Division of Bacterial Diseases, National Cen ter for Immunization and Respiratory Diseases, Centers for Disease Control and Prevention (CDC). MMWR Re comm Rep 2010;59:1–36.

- If intraamniotic infection is suspected during labor, initiation of a broad-spectrum antibiotic regimen that also covers GBS is recommended. PCN or cefazolin as a single agent in this setting can then be discontinued.
- For patients who present with preterm premature rupture of membranes and are receiving intravenous latency antibiotics, that regimen should cover GBS. A GBS

test swab should be collected before starting antibiotics, as it can help guide therapy if the patient remains undelivered for > 5 weeks.

Patients with GBS colonization in a prior pregnancy have been shown to have a 50% likelihood of being colonized in a subsequent pregnancy.[30] As a result, patients presenting in labor at term with unknown GBS status can be considered to receive IAP based on those data.[4]

Group B Streptococcus Bacteriuria

Patients with GBS bacteriuria at any colony count during pregnancy should be assumed to have a higher level of GBS colonization and should receive IAP[31] (**Box 1**). As with any other pathogenic bacteria, GBS bacteriuria at a colony count $<10^5$ CFUs, does not itself need to be acutely treated.

Prenatal antibiotics for other indications do not completely eradicate GBS colonization and it is common to have recolonization after a course of antibiotics.[32] Therefore, treatment of subthreshold bacteriuria for GBS "prevention" purposes before delivery is neither effective nor indicated.

INTRAPARTUM ANTIBIOTIC PROPHYLAXIS
Antibiotic Prophylaxis Agents

Antibiotic prophylaxis acts to serve two goals

1. Decreasing incidence of neonatal GBS colonization via adequate maternal drug levels.
2. Reducing the risk of neonatal sepsis via adequate fetal and newborn drug levels.

Box 1
Antepartum GBS bacteriuria and intrapartum prophylaxis key points

- Group B streptococcus (GBS) bacteriuria at any concentration identified in pregnancy represents heavy maternal vaginal-rectal colonization and indicates the need for intrapartum antibiotic prophylaxis without the need for a subsequent GBS screening vaginal-rectal culture

- GBS bacteriuria at levels of 10^5 colony-forming units (CFUs)/mL or greater, whether asymptomatic or symptomatic, warrants acute treatment as well as need for intrapartum antibiotic prophylaxis

- Identification of asymptomatic GBS bacteriuria during pregnancy at a level less than 10^5 CFUs/mL does not require maternal antibiotic therapy during the antepartum period however is an indication for intrapartum antibiotic prophylaxis

- Any urine culture sent for laboratory evaluation during pregnancy should be marked as being that of a pregnant patient

- In patients who have a reported penicillin allergy, laboratory requisitions for antepartum urine cultures should be marked for the laboratory to be aware of the allergy and ensure that GBS isolates will be appropriately tested for clindamycin susceptibility

- Clindamycin susceptibility results reported on GBS-positive urine cultures should only be used to guide antibiotic choice for intrapartum antibiotic prophylaxis. Clindamycin is not recommended as a treatment agent for urinary tract infections as it is poorly concentrated in urine, metabolized primarily by the liver, and intended to mainly treat bloodstream and soft tissue infections.

From Prevention of Group B Streptococcal Early-Onset Disease in Newborns: ACOG Committee Opinion, Number 797 [published correction appears in Obstet Gynecol. 2020 Apr;135(4):978-979]. Obstet Gynecol. 2020;135(2):e51-e72.

The algorithm for the use of IAP regimens to prevent GBS infection in newborns is pictured in **Table 1**.

The best first agent of choice for GBS antibiotic prophylaxis is intravenous PCN G. Although ampicillin is an acceptable alternative if PCN is unavailable, PCN is preferred over other agents due to its narrower, more targeted antimicrobial coverage of gram-positive bacteria and its lower likelihood of inducing resistance in other organisms, particularly *Escherichia coli*. Resistant *E coli* have been isolated from newborns whose mothers received less than 24 h of ampicillin during labor.[33]

Recommended dosages for both PCN and ampicillin (**Fig. 1**) have been shown to achieve adequate minimum inhibitory concentrations (MICs) in both fetal blood and amniotic fluid, with minimal risk of maternal toxicity. PCN G administered to the mother readily crosses the placenta, reaching peak cord blood concentrations by 1 h and rapidly declining by 4 h, reflecting elimination of the antibiotic by the fetal kidney into amniotic fluid.[34] Ampicillin has been detected in cord blood within 30 min and in amniotic fluid within 45 min of administration to the mother.[35]

Management in Patients with Penicillin Allergies

For a GBS-colonized pregnant patient with a reported PCN allergy, the two most important assessments are.

1. The nature of the PCN allergy and risk of a severe reaction (**Table 2**).
2. The susceptibility of the GBS isolate to clindamycin.[36,37]

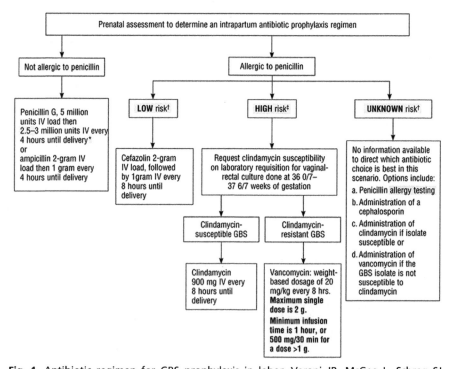

Fig. 1. Antibiotic regimen for GBS prophylaxis in labor. Verani JR, McGee L, Schrag SJ. Prevention of perinatal group B streptococcal disease—revised guidelines from CDC, 2010. Division of Bacterial Diseases, National Cen ter for Immunization and Respiratory Diseases, Centers for Disease Control and Prevention (CDC). MMWR Re comm Rep 2010;59:1–36.

Table 2
Penicillin allergy risk stratification

Risk	Definition
Low risk	Nonspecific symptoms unlikely to be allergic (gastrointestinal distress, headaches, yeast vaginitis)
	Nonurticarial maculopapular (morbilliform) rash without systemic symptoms[a]
	Pruritus without rash
	Family history of penicillin allergy but no personal history
	Patient reports but has no recollection of symptoms or treatment
High risk	High risk for anaphylaxis: A history suggestive of an IgE-mediated event[b]: Pruritic rash, urticaria (hives), immediate flushing, hypotension, angioedema, respiratory distress or anaphylaxis[c]
	Recurrent reactions, reaction to multiple beta-lactam antibiotics, or positive penicillin allergy test
	High risk for severe non-IgE-mediated reaction: Severe rare delayed-onset cutaneous or systemic reactions, such as eosinophilia and systemic symptoms/drug-induced hypersensitivity syndrome, Stevens–Johnson syndrome, or toxic epidermal necrolysis[d]

[a] This rash typically occurs several days after initial exposure and is limited to the skin (mucous membranes, palm, and soles are not involved). May be mildly pruritic but not urticarial.
[b] Anaphylactic reactions are IgE mediated and typically occur within 1 to 6 h after exposure to penicillin.
[c] Some institutions have performed penicillin allergy testing in pregnant women with a history suggestive an IgE-mediated event (classified by some experts as a moderate risk of anaphylaxis): urticaria (hives), isolated urticaria occurring greater than 10 y prior, or intense pruritic rash. Penicillin allergy testing can be achieved in these situations through referral to an allergy and immunology specialist.
[d] Severe rare delayed-onset reactions, such as eosinophilia and systemic symptoms/drug-induced hypersensitivity syndrome, Stevens-Johnson syndrome, or toxic epidermal necrolysis are T-cell mediated and typically occur days to weeks after initiation of antibiotic treatment. Some experts consider these a contraindication to standard penicillin allergy testing.
From Prevention of Group B Streptococcal Early-Onset Disease in Newborns: ACOG Committee Opinion, Number 797 [published correction appears in Obstet Gynecol. 2020 Apr;135(4):978-979]. Obstet Gynecol. 2020;135(2):e51-e72.

PCN allergy testing is considered safe in pregnancy and should be discussed with and offered to all patients who report a PCN allergy.[38] Confirming the absence of a type I hypersensitivity reaction would allow use of the first-line agent PCN and positively impact the patient's medical management beyond pregnancy as well.[38]

Recent reviews have advised that most persons with a reported PCN allergy are actually PCN tolerant.[38,39] Approximately 80% to 90% of persons who report a history of PCN allergy are not truly allergic because the sensitization is lost over time or the original reaction was not related to PCN.[40,41]

Because severe allergic reactions are uncommon, cephalosporins (cefazolin) are recommended for women whose reported PCN allergy is low risk for anaphylaxis or of uncertain severity. In contrast to older studies reporting higher rates, more recent reports, based on results from skin allergy testing, estimated that allergic reactions occur in only 4.3% of patients with PCN allergy when administered first-generation and second-generation cephalosporins and in less than 1% of patients administered third-generation and fourth-generation cephalosporins.[42] Although cefazolin is a first-generation cephalosporin, it has a unique configuration and very low cross-reactivity with PCN.[43]

For patients with an allergy with high risk of anaphylaxis or severe rare delayed-onset reaction, the GBS isolate should be evaluated for clindamycin susceptibility via D-zone testing, which indicates the presence of inducible resistance from macrolides including erythromycin. If the isolate is susceptible to both clindamycin and erythromycin, the patient should receive clindamycin.[44,45] This susceptibility testing is very important, as rates of GBS resistance to clindamycin have continued to rise over the past decade, and most recently have been reported to range from 40% to 68% globally.[46–48]

For patients with a high-risk PCN allergy and whose GBS isolate is not susceptible to clindamycin, intravenous vancomycin should be administered.[49,50] The recommended dosing for IAP with vancomycin, as outlined in the current ACOG guidelines, is weight-based, at 20 mg/kg every 8 h, with a maximum of 2 g per dose. Vancomycin infusions should ideally be run over at least 1 h to minimize flushing, potentially 2 h for doses higher than 1 g.

This revised dosing schedule is similar to the manner in which vancomycin dosing is routinely calculated for most nonobstetric populations.[51–53] It has also been shown to have improved placental transfer and better therapeutic levels in neonatal blood samples compared with the prior dosing of 1 g every 12 h.[49,50]

Baseline testing consisting of a serum creatinine level and estimated creatinine clearance is recommended before starting vancomycin given the renal clearance of the drug. Still, the short course for which vancomycin would be used for GBS prophylaxis would not be expected to have significant renal side effects, in contrast to its use for longer time periods in managing more serious adult infections.[54]

INTRAPARTUM OBSTETRIC MANAGEMENT CONSIDERATIONS
Duration of Antibiotic Prophylaxis

Studies evaluating the ideal time interval for beta-lactam prophylaxis for GBS showed that maternal antibiotic prophylaxis given at least 4 h before birth to be most effective, compared with intervals started under 4 h before birth.[55]

Still, antibiotic administration starting at least 2 h before delivery has been shown to significantly reduce vaginal GBS colony counts and frequency of clinical neonatal sepsis.[56] Longer duration of intrapartum antibiotic usage reduced the risks for both neonatal sepsis evaluation and empiric neonatal antibiotic administration in a dose-response manner: 1.6% in cases where antibiotics were given less than 2 h before delivery, 0.9% between 2 and 4 h, and 0.4% for 4 h or greater.[56]

Obstetric interventions as deemed medically necessary should not be delayed for the purpose of antibiotic timing before delivery. These interventions include initiation of oxytocin, artificial rupture of membranes, or planned cesarean delivery.

Obstetric Procedures

There is overall insufficient high-quality research to support or discourage various obstetric procedures in patients with GBS colonization in labor.

Membrane sweeping (or stripping) has been performed to potentially reduce duration of pregnancy and likelihood of late-term gestation.[57] Evidence is limited regarding risk of bacterial seeding with membrane sweeping in GBS-colonized patients and is limited to case reports or anecdotal evidence. One prospective cohort study did not find an increased risk of clinical indicators for neonatal sepsis or maternal infection with membrane stripping in GBS-positive patients.[58]

Similarly, there is a paucity of data, and therefore no formal recommendation on timing of IAP in patients colonized with GBS undergoing mechanical cervical ripening, and best clinical judgment should be used.

Artificial rupture of membranes in patients colonized with GBS has not been associated with an increased risk of GBS EOD when IAP is given.[59] Although augmentation of labor should be performed as clinically indicated, consideration can be given to postponing amniotomy or administration of oxytocin as clinically allowable to ensure a full 4 h of antibiotic administration before delivery.

SUMMARY

The most effective strategy to date for reducing GBS EOD entails universal antenatal GBS screening and IAP as appropriate and guided by screening results. If NAAT is used as primary antenatal GBS screening, clindamycin susceptibility testing for PCN allergic patients should be incorporated and reported.

Hospital systems should designate groups or committees of specialty experts to ensure appropriate GBS screening and collection, proper use of antibiotics, and consistent education on these topics and practices. Health agencies should maintain surveillance systems to monitor incidence of GBS EOD, emergence of resistant organisms, and any maternal or neonatal complications of widespread antibiotic usage including severe allergic reactions and effect on the pediatric microbiome.

Overall, a combination of efforts should be used to minimize the risk of GBS EOD in a safe and sustainable manner.

CLINICS CARE POINTS

- Intravenous intrapartum antibiotic prophylaxis (IAP) has been shown to be effective for the prevention of GBS early-onset disease (EOD) in patients with confirmed GBS colonization or intrapartum risk factors for colonization.

- All pregnant patients should undergo antepartum GBS screening between 36 0/7 and 37 6/7 weeks of gestation, regardless of planned mode of birth.

- Patients with GBS bacteriuria or history of newborn with GBS disease should automatically receive IAP and can defer screening.

- Patients with a positive GBS vaginal-rectal culture at any point in the pregnancy should receive IAP, with the exception of those undergoing a pre-labor cesarean delivery with intact membranes.

- Patients who undergo a cesarean delivery before the onset of labor and with intact membranes do not require GBS antibiotic prophylaxis.

- Patients with plan for scheduled cesarean delivery should still receive GBS screening in the case that they enter labor or have ruptured membranes before their cesarean delivery, in which case they should receive antibiotic prophylaxis.

- If GBS status is unknown at the time of labor onset, IAP should be administered in the setting of the following risk factors for GBS EOD: risk of preterm birth, preterm prelabor rupture of membranes, rupture of membranes for 18 or more hours at term, or intrapartum fever (temperature 100.4°F [38°C] or higher).

- If intraamniotic infection is suspected, broad-spectrum antibiotic therapy that includes GBS coverage should be initiated.

- If GBS status is unknown at term at the time of labor onset and the patient has a history of GBS colonization in a prior pregnancy, it is reasonable to offer IAP as there is up to 50% risk of GBS colonization recurrence and thus increased risk of GBS EOD.

- The antibiotic of choice for GBS prophylaxis is intravenous penicillin; intravenous ampicillin is an acceptable alternative.

- Patients with low-risk penicillin allergy or an allergy of unknown severity can receive first-generation cephalosporins, such as cefazolin.

- Patients with high-risk penicillin allergies should have their GBS isolate evaluated for clindamycin susceptibility via ᴅ-zone testing and can receive clindamycin if the isolate is susceptible.
- Patients with high-risk penicillin allergies and with GBS isolates not susceptible to clindamycin should receive intravenous vancomycin at weight-based dosing (20 mg/kg intravenously every 8 h, up to maximum 2 g per dose) and have baseline renal function evaluated.
- Patients who report a history of penicillin allergy should undergo penicillin allergy testing, which is safe in pregnancy.
- Obstetric interventions, including planned cesarean delivery, artificial rupture of membranes, and initiation of oxytocin, should not be delayed solely to provide the ideal 4 h of antibiotic coverage before birth.

DISCLOSURE

The authors report no conflict of interest.

REFERENCES

1. Schrag SJ, Verani JR. Intrapartum antibiotic prophylaxis for the prevention of perinatal group B streptococcal disease: experience in the United States and implications for a potential group B streptococcal vaccine. Vaccine 2013;31(suppl 4):D20–6.
2. Boyer KM, Gadzala CA, Burd LI, et al. Selective intrapartum chemoprophylaxis of neonatal group B streptococcal early-onset disease. I. Epidemiologic rationale. J Infect Dis 1983;148:795–801.
3. Nanduri SA, Petit S, Smelser C, et al. Epidemiology of Invasive Early-Onset and Late-Onset Group B Streptococcal Disease in the United States, 2006 to 2015: Multistate Laboratory and Population-Based Surveillance. JAMA Pediatr 2019; 173(3):224–33.
4. Prevention of Group B. Streptococcal Early-Onset Disease in Newborns: ACOG Committee Opinion, Number 797. Obstet Gynecol 2020 Feb;135(2):e51–72.
5. Anthony BF, Okada DM, Hobel CJ. Epidemiology of group B Streptococcus: longitudinal observations during pregnancy. J Infect Dis 1978;137:524–30.
6. Anthony BF, Okada DM, Hobel CJ. Epidemiology of the group B streptococcus: maternal and nosocomial sources for infant acquisitions. J Pediatr 1979;95: 431–6.
7. Phares CR, Lynfield R, Farley MM, et al. Epidemiology of invasive group B streptococcal disease in the United States, 1999–2005. Active Bacterial Core surveillance/Emerging Infections Program Network. JAMA 2008;299:2056–65.
8. Le Doare K, Heath PT. An overview of global GBS epidemiology. Vaccine 2013; 31(suppl 4):D7–12.
9. Schrag SJ, Farley MM, Petit S, et al. Epidemiology of invasive early-onset neonatal sepsis, 2005 to 2014. Pediatrics 2016;138:e20162013.
10. Berardi A, Rossi C, Lugli L, et al. Group B streptococcus late-onset disease: 2003–2010. GBS Prevention Working Group, Emilia-Romagna. Pediatrics 2013; 131:e361–8.
11. Russell NJ, Seale AC, O'Sullivan C, et al. Risk of early-onset neonatal group B streptococcal disease with maternal colonization worldwide: systematic review and meta-analyses. Clin Infect Dis 2017;65:S152–9.

12. Creti R, Imperi M, Berardi A, et al. Neonatal group B streptococcus infections: prevention strategies, clinical and microbiologic characteristics in 7 years of surveillance. Italian Neonatal GBS Infections Working Group. Pediatr Infect Dis J 2017;36:256–62.

13. Campbell JR, Hillier SL, Krohn MA, et al. Group B streptococcal colonization and serotype-specific immunity in pregnant women at delivery. Obstet Gynecol 2000; 96:498–503.

14. Regan JA, Klebanoff MA, Nugent RP. The epidemiology of group B streptococcal colonization in pregnancy. Vaginal Infections and Prematurity Study Group. Obstet Gynecol 1991;77:604–10.

15. Seale AC, Bianchi-Jassir F, Russell NJ, et al. Estimates of the burden of group B streptococcal disease worldwide for pregnant women, stillbirths, and children. Clin Infect Dis 2017;65:S200–19.

16. Muller AE, Oostvogel PM, Steegers EA, et al. Morbidity related to maternal group B streptococcal infections. Acta Obstet Gynecol Scand 2006;85:1027–37.

17. Bianchi-Jassir F, Seale AC, Kohli-Lynch M, et al. Preterm birth associated with group B streptococcus maternal colonization worldwide: systematic review and meta-analyses. Clin Infect Dis 2017;65:S133–42.

18. Schuchat A, Deaver-Robinson K, Plikaytis BD, et al. Multistate case–control study of maternal risk factors for neonatal group B streptococcal disease. The Active Surveillance Study Group. Pediatr Infect Dis J 1994;13:623–9.

19. Kessous R, Weintraub AY, Sergienko R, et al. Bacteriuria with group-B streptococcus: is it a risk factor for adverse pregnancy outcomes? J Matern Fetal Neonatal Med 2012;25:1983 – 6.

20. Weeks JW, Myers SR, Lasher L, et al. Persistence of penicillin G benzathine in pregnant group B streptococcus carriers. Obstet Gynecol 1997;90:240–3.

21. Ohlsson A, Shah VS, Stade BC. Vaginal chlorhexidine during labour to prevent early-onset neonatal group B streptococcal infection. Cochrane Database Syst Rev 2014;12:CD003520.

22. Boyer KM, Gadzala CA, Kelly PD, et al. Selective intrapartum chemoprophylaxis of neonatal group B streptococcal early-onset disease. II. Predictive value of prenatal cultures. J Infect Dis 1983;148:802–9.

23. Yancey MK, Schuchat A, Brown LK, et al. The accuracy of late antenatal screening cultures in predicting genital group B streptococcal colonization at delivery. Obstet Gynecol 1996;88:811–5.

24. Philipson EH, Palermino DA, Robinson A. Enhanced antenatal detection of group B streptococcus colonization. Obstet Gynecol 1995;85:437–9.

25. Mercer BM, Taylor MC, Fricke JL, et al. The accuracy and patient preference for self-collected group B streptococcus cultures. Am J Obstet Gynecol 1995;173: 1325–8.

26. Curry A, Bookless G, Donaldson K, et al. Evaluation of hibergene loop-mediated isothermal amplification assay for detection of group B streptococcus in rectovaginal swabs: a prospective diagnostic accuracy study. Clin Microbiol Infect 2018;24:1066–9.

27. Alfa MJ, Sepehri S, De Gagne P, et al. Real-time PCR assay provides reliable assessment of intrapartum carriage of group B Streptococcus. J Clin Microbiol 2010;48:3095–9.

28. Hakansson S, Axemo P, Bremme K, et al. Group B streptococcal carriage in Sweden: a national study on risk factors for mother and infant colonisation. Swedish Working Group For The Prevention of Perinatal Group B Streptococcal Infections. Acta Obstet Gynecol Scand 2008;87:50–8.

29. Use of prophylactic antibiotics in labor and delivery. ACOG Practice Bulletin No. 199. American College of Obstetricians and Gynecologists. Obstet Gynecol 2018;132:e103–19.

30. Turrentine MA, Colicchia LC, Hirsch E, et al. Efficiency of screening for the recurrence of antenatal group B streptococcus colonization in a subsequent pregnancy: a systematic review and meta-analysis with independent patient data. Am J Perinatol 2016;33:510–7.

31. Perez-Moreno MO, Pico-Plana E, Grande-Armas J, et al. Group B streptococcal bacteriuria during pregnancy as a risk factor for maternal intrapartum colonization: a prospective cohort study. J Med Microbiol 2017;66:454–60.

32. Baecher L, Grobman W. Prenatal antibiotic treatment does not decrease group B streptococcus colonization at delivery. Int J Gynaecol Obstet 2008;101:125–8.

33. Flannery DD, Akinboyo IC, Mukhopadhyay S, et al. Antibiotic Susceptibility of Escherichia coli Among Infants Admitted to Neonatal Intensive Care Units Across the US From 2009 to 2017. JAMA Pediatr 2021;175(2):168–75.

34. Barber EL, Zhao G, Buhimschi IA, et al. Duration of intrapartum prophylaxis and concentration of penicillin G in fetal serum at delivery. Obstet Gynecol 2008;112:265–7.

35. Yow MD, Mason EO, Leeds LJ, et al. Ampicillin prevents intrapartum transmission of group B streptococcus. JAMA 1979;241:1245–7.

36. Paccione KA, Wiesenfeld HC. Guideline adherence for intrapartum group B streptococci prophylaxis in penicillin-allergic patients. Infect Dis Obstet Gynecol 2013;2013:917304.

37. Briody VA, Albright CM, Has P, et al. Use of cefazolin for group B streptococci prophylaxis in women reporting a penicillin allergy without anaphylaxis. Obstet Gynecol 2016;127:577–83.

38. Shenoy ES, Macy E, Rowe T, et al. Evaluation and management of penicillin allergy: a review. JAMA 2019;321:188–99.

39. Turrentine MA, King T, Silverman NS. Penicillin allergy in pregnancy: Moving from "rash" decisions to accurate diagnosis. Clinical Expert Series. Obstet Gynecol 2020;135:401–8.

40. Drug allergy: an updated practice parameter. Joint Task Force on Practice Parameters, American Academy of Allergy, Asthma and Immunology, American College of Allergy, Asthma and Immunology, Joint Council of Allergy, Asthma and Immunology. Ann Allergy Asthma Immunol 2010;105:259–73.

41. Macy E, Vyles D. Who needs penicillin allergy testing? Ann Allergy Asthma Immunol 2018;121:523–9.

42. Kelkar PS, Li JT. Cephalosporin allergy. N Engl J Med 2001;345:804–9.

43. Lee QU. Use of cephalosporins in patients with immediate penicillin hypersensitivity: cross-reactivity revisited. Hong Kong Med J 2014;20:428–36.

44. Woods CR. Macrolide-inducible resistance to clindamycin and the D-est. Pediatr Infect Dis J 2009;28:1115–8.

45. Verani JR, McGee L, Schrag SJ. Prevention of perinatal group B streptococcal disease: revised guidelines from CDC, 2010. Division of Bacterial Diseases, National Center for Immunization ad Respiratory Diseases, Centers for Disease Control and Prevention (CDC). MMWR Recomm Rep (Morb Mortal Wkly Rep) 2010;59(RR-10):1–36.

46. Ma A, Thompson LA, Corsiatto T, et al. Epidemiological Characterization of Group B Streptococcus Infections in Alberta, Canada: An Update from 2014 to 2020. Microbiol Spectr 2021;17:e0128321.

47. Ge Y, Pan F, Bai R, et al. Prevalence of group B streptococcus colonization in pregnant women in Jiangsu, East China. BMC Infect Dis 2021;21(1):1–5.
48. Clindamycin-Resistant Group B. Streptococcus. Center for Disease Control. Available at: https://www.cdc.gov/drugresistance/pdf/threats-report/gbs-508.pdf. Accessed January 2, 2023.
49. Onwuchuruba CN, Towers CV, Howard BC, et al. Transplacental passage of vancomycin from mother to neonate. Am J Obstet Gynecol 2014;210:352, e1– 4.
50. Towers CV, Weitz B. Transplacental passage of vancomycin. J Matern Fetal Neonatal Med 2018;31:1021–4.
51. Rybak M, Lomaestro B, Rotschafer JC, et al. Therapeutic monitoring of vancomycin in adult patients: a consensus review of the American Society of Health-System Pharmacists, the Infectious Diseases Society of America, and the Society of Infectious Diseases Pharmacists. Am J Health Syst Pharm 2009;66:82–98.
52. Koliha K, Falk J, Patel R, et al. Comparative evaluation of pharmacist-managed vancomycin dosing in a community hospital following implementation of a system-wide vancomycin dosing guideline. J Pharm Pharmacol 2017;5:607–15.
53. Liu C, Bayer A, Cosgrove SE, et al. Clinical practice guidelines by the Infectious Diseases Society of America for the treatment of methicillin-resistant Staphylococcus aureus infections in adults and children. Infectious Diseases Society of America. Clin Infect Dis 2011;52:18–55.
54. Rybak MJ. The pharmacokinetic and pharmacodynamic properties of vancomycin. Clin Infect Dis 2006;42(suppl 1):S35–9.
55. Fairlie T, Zell ER, Schrag S. Effectiveness of intrapartum antibiotic prophylaxis for prevention of early-onset group B streptococcal disease. Obstet Gynecol 2013; 121:570–7.
56. Turrentine MA, Greisinger AJ, Brown KS, et al. Duration of intrapartum antibiotics for group B streptococcus on the diagnosis of clinical neonatal sepsis. Infect Dis Obstet Gynecol 2013;2013:525878.
57. Boulvain M, Stan CM, Irion O. Membrane sweeping for induction of labour. Cochrane Database Syst Rev 2005;2:CD000451.
58. Kabiri D, Hants Y, Yarkoni TR, et al. Antepartum membrane stripping in GBS carriers, is it safe? (the STRIP-G Study). PLoS One 2015;10:e0145905.
59. Adair CE, Kowalsky L, Quon H, et al. Risk factors for early-onset group B streptococcal disease in neonates: a population-based case-control study. CMAJ (Can Med Assoc J) 2003;169:198–203.

Human Immunodeficiency Virus in Pregnancy

Annie M. Dude, MD, PhD*, Maura Jones, MD, Tenisha Wilson, MD, PhD

KEYWORDS

- Human immunodeficiency virus • Pregnancy • Antiretroviral therapy
- Perinatal transmission

KEY POINTS

- All patients should be offered the opportunity for opt-out testing for human immunodeficiency virus (HIV) during pregnancy.
- Maternal antiretroviral therapy is key for optimizing maternal health and preventing perinatal transmission for patients living with HIV.
- With appropriate care during the prepregnancy, antepartum, intrapartum, and postpartum periods, the risk for perinatal transmission of HIV is less than 1%.

BACKGROUND

Human immunodeficiency virus (HIV) infection in pregnant people remains a public health concern in the United States as well as worldwide. An estimated 34,800 people in the United States received a diagnosis of HIV in 2019; of these, about 22% were in patients identified as female at birth.[1] Approximately 5000 people living with HIV give birth in the United States each year.[2]

Perinatal transmission of HIV can occur during the antepartum, intrapartum, and postpartum periods. The rate of perinatal transmission is between 15% and 45% when patients do not receive appropriate therapies during these periods, including antiretroviral therapy (ART), intrapartum prophylaxis (usually zidovudine), and neonatal prophylaxis.[3] This rate can be reduced to less than 1% with these and other measures.[4,5] Perinatal transmission in the United States and dependent areas has declined by more than 95% since the early 1990s.[6] Yet, perinatal transmission persists between 2011 and 2016, an estimated 99 cases of vertical transmission occurred in the United States.[7] These cases of perinatal transmission in the United States are usually associated with lack of timely diagnosis, lack of prenatal care, and/or lack of ART.

Division of Maternal-Fetal Medicine, Department of Obstetrics & Gynecology, University of North Carolina at Chapel Hill, Chapel Hill, NC, USA
* Corresponding author. 3010 Old Clinic Building, Campus Box 7570, Chapel Hill, NC 27599.
E-mail address: annie_dude@med.unc.edu

Obstet Gynecol Clin N Am 50 (2023) 389–399
https://doi.org/10.1016/j.ogc.2023.02.010
0889-8545/23/© 2023 Elsevier Inc. All rights reserved.

obgyn.theclinics.com

HIV infection also poses health risks to pregnant patients, including increased risk of opportunistic infections, as CD4 T-lymphocyte counts fall during pregnancy,[8] increased risk of gestational diabetes (as impaired glucose metabolism is associated with certain protease inhibitors),[9] and increased risk of obstetric severe maternal morbidity and mortality.[10,11] These risks can be alleviated with ART and other measures.

The goal of this document is to describe how to screen for HIV in pregnancy, how to optimize care for patients living with HIV, and how to reduce the risk of perinatal transmission during the prepregnancy, antepartum, intrapartum, and postpartum periods.

DISCUSSION

Human Immunodeficiency Virus Testing in Pregnancy

The Centers for Disease Control and Prevention (CDC), the United States Preventative Services Task Force, and the American College of Obstetricians and Gynecologists (ACOG) all recommend universal, opt-out testing for HIV at least one time during pregnancy, ideally in the first trimester or at the first prenatal care visit.[12–14] "Opt-out" indicates that patients should be informed that an HIV test is part of routine obstetric care and that they will be tested unless they specifically decline the test.[14] Studies show this method results in higher percentages of patients being tested for HIV than "opt-in" testing, where patients are tested only if they specifically give verbal or written consent.[15] ACOG also recommends repeat third trimester testing for patients who are at high risk of HIV transmission based on local prevalence or patient symptoms consistent with acute HIV infection, such as fever, lymphadenopathy, myalgias, and others.[12] Third trimester HIV testing is also required by law in several states.[16] Finally, for patients who were not tested during routine prenatal care or for whom HIV status is otherwise unknown, ACOG recommends rapid testing when presenting for delivery or immediately postpartum using an opt-out approach.[12] When a person's HIV status remains unknown following delivery, testing of the newborn is recommended.[14]

Initial screening tests indicating an HIV infection use antigen/antibody testing. The CDC currently recommends a "fourth generation" test with both antibodies (IgG and IgM) as well as the p24 antigen. These fourth-generation tests allow for earlier detection (within 10 days of infection) than earlier iterations of antibody-only tests, have 99% sensitivity, and have 99% specificity as well.[17] These tests must be confirmed with antibody differentiation assays that distinguish between HIV-1 and HIV-2. If patients test negative or indeterminate for both HIV-1 and HIV-2 with these differentiation assays, confirmation with a nucleic acid test is recommended.[18] See **Fig. 1** for the current CDC testing algorithm.

Prepregnancy Care for Patients Living with Human Immunodeficiency Virus

Before pregnancy, there are a number of actions patients and clinicians can undertake to improve a pregnant person's health during pregnancy, decrease the chances of perinatal transmission, and decrease the chances of transmission to an uninfected partner. Foundational to improving health for the potentially pregnant person and to avoid transmission is treatment with ART to achieve an undetectable viral load, which greatly reduces the risk of either sexual transmission while attempting conception or perinatal transmission.[19] Although beyond the scope of this document, all patients living with HIV who have a serodiscordant partner (ie, a partner that is HIV-negative) should discuss the possibility of pre-exposure prophylaxis, or PrEP. In brief, PrEP in the context of pregnancy consists of antiretrovirals taken by HIV seronegative sexual

Recommended Laboratory HIV Testing Algorithm for Serum or Plasma Specimens

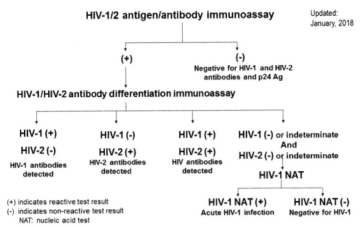

Fig. 1. CDC testing algorithm for HIV in pregnancy. (*From* Centers for Disease Control and Prevention (CDC). 2018 Quick reference guide: Recommended laboratory HIV testing algorithm for serum or plasma specimens. Published June 2014, updated January 2018. Available at https://stacks.cdc.gov/view/cdc/50872 and https://www.cdc.gov/hiv/pdf/guidelines_testing_recommendedlabtestingalgorithm.pdf.)

partners of patients living with HIV while having condomless intercourse with the goal of becoming pregnant. If patients living with HIV have an undetectable viral load, it is unclear whether there is an additional benefit in terms of risk reduction for their partners to take PreP.[20]

Several prepregnancy vaccinations are recommended: for those with CD4 counts greater than 200 cells per cubic millimeter, varicella and rubella should be given if patients are not already immune. All patients living with HIV should be vaccinated against influenza, pneumococcus, the human papilloma virus, hepatitis B, hepatitis A, severe acute respiratory syndrome coronavirus 2, and Tdap.[21]

In the prepregnancy period and throughout pregnancy, patients with CD4 T-lymphocyte counts below certain thresholds may need to be initiated on prophylactic medications to protect against opportunistic infections. A list of these infections and prophylactic medications can be found in **Table 1**.

Antepartum Care for Patients Living with Human Immunodeficiency Virus

Pregnant persons should begin ART as early as possible to improve their health outcomes, regardless of CD4 counts or viral load. In general, if a person who becomes pregnant is on a regimen with a sustained undetectable viral load, that regimen should be continued. The same regimens that are recommended for the treatment of nonpregnant adults should be used in pregnant adults. Important considerations in selecting a regimen include the risks and benefits of the medications for each person who becomes pregnant, previous experience with ART regimens, compliance, and pill aversions. For persons who become pregnant and are not on ART, initiation is recommended as soon as possible after HIV infection is diagnosed.

There are several considerations regarding ART use specific to pregnancy. For people with nausea and vomiting of pregnancy, proactive treatment with antiemetics is recommended. The increased volume of distribution and glomerular filtration rate

Table 1
Prophylaxis for common opportunistic infections in patients living with human immunodeficiency virus

CD4 Count	Notes	Opportunistic Infection	Prophylactic Medication
<200	CD4 < 200 OR CD < 14%	*Pneumocystis jirovecii* Pneumonia	TMP-SMX 1 tablet double strength by mouth daily
<150	Occupational exposures or live in a community with a high endemic rate (>10 cases histoplasma/100 patient y)	Histoplasma	Itraconazole 200 mg by mouth daily
<100		*Toxoplasma gondii*	TMX-SMX one tablet double strength by mouth daily
<50	Not recommended with immediate initiation of ART to avoid immune reconstitution	MAC Mycobacterium avium complex disease	Azithromycin 1200 mg by mouth once weekly Or clarithromycin 500 mg by mouth twice per d Or Azithromycin 600 mg by mouth twice weekly

changes medication pharmacokinetics, and several drugs may have subtherapeutic levels in the third trimester. In patients who have a viral load greater than 500 copies/mL, ART drug resistance genotype evaluation should be performed to ensure optimal ART selection before starting ART or modifying regimens. However, ART initiation should not be delayed before genotype results are available.

There are a number of laboratory tests that should be ordered in addition to standard prenatal laboratories for patients living with HIV and on ART. A list of these laboratories can be found in **Table 2**.

In terms of prenatal diagnosis, pregnant people living with HIV should be offered genetic counseling, including options of noninvasive and invasive testing. Recent studies indicate that for pregnant persons on ART with a sustained undetectable viral load, HIV transmission rates with chorionic villus sampling and amniocentesis are not increased from baseline.[22] Patients living with HIV do not have a higher risk of birth defects than the general population, even when on ART.[23–25] People living with HIV should be offered routine first and second trimester anatomy scans as any other pregnant person, and diagnostic testing should not be withheld.

Intrapartum Care for Patients Living with Human Immunodeficiency Virus

Pregnant patients with HIV should have viral loads reassessed between 34 to 36 weeks in anticipation of delivery to guide recommendations and management. Patients should be counseled regarding mode of delivery based on the results of this test.

Management in Those with Viral Loads Greater than 1000 Copies/mL

Patients with unknown viral loads or viral loads greater than 1000 should be counseled on the benefits of cesarean delivery on the risk of vertical transmission. A 1999 randomized controlled trial by the European Mode of Delivery Collaboration demonstrated a vertical transmission rate of 2% for those undergoing scheduled cesarean

Table 2
Laboratory tests in the context of human immunodeficiency virus

Laboratory test	Time Period					
	Before Pregnancy	On Entry to Prenatal Care	Every Trimester	Every Month	34-36 wk	Other
HIV viral load	X	X	X	X[c]	X	
CD4 T-lymphocyte count	X	X		X[d]		
Complete blood count	X	X	X			
Liver and kidney function tests	X	X	X			
Antiretroviral drug resistance (genotype) panel	X					
G6PD[a] and HLA-B*5701[b]	X					
Toxoplasmosis IgG	X					
Hepatitis A, B, and C screening		X				
Sexually transmitted infection screening		X				
Tuberculosis screening	X					

[a] If positive, do not use abacavir for ART.
[b] If G6PD deficiency is present, then avoid trimethoprim/sulfamethoxazole for *Pneumocystis jirovecii* prophylaxis.
[c] If viral RNA remains detectable, then check viral loads every month.
[d] For individuals who have been on ART less than 2 y, individuals with CD4 counts lower than 300 cells/mm^3, individuals with detectable viral loads, and in individuals who have inconsistent adherence to ART.

section compared with a rate of 10% for those undergoing other modes of delivery.[26] Given this, the benefit of scheduling a cesarean delivery at 38 weeks or otherwise before the onset of labor or rupture of membranes should be included in counseling and offered. For those undergoing scheduled cesarean, intravenous zidovudine should be administered at least 3 hours before the scheduled cesarean delivery.[27]

For those who present in labor or with rupture of membranes (before cesarean), zidovudine should be initiated on presentation. The Mothers' and Infants' Cohort Study examined that the relationship between rupture of membranes and vertical transmission of HIV and found that rupture for $\geq$ 4 hours was associated with a significantly higher rate of transmission, regardless of the duration of labor or mode of delivery.[28] A 2001 meta-analysis by the International Perinatal HIV Group looked at over 4000 deliveries with rupture of membranes for $\leq$ 24 hours and found the risk of vertical transmission increased approximately 2% per hour in those with HIV and even more so in those with AIDS.[29] Therefore, the delivery plan should be individualized, as the benefit of a cesarean in reducing the risk of perinatal transmission may not persist if membranes have been ruptured for a significant length of time.

Management in Those with Viral Loads Less than 1000 Copies/mL

In those with viral loads less than 1000 on ART, the risk of transmission is low, regardless of the mode of delivery or duration of membrane rupture. Therefore, cesarean is not routinely recommended in this population and should be reserved for the standard obstetric indications, with delivery timing according to the obstetric indication.[27,30] Briand and colleagues reviewed the mode of delivery from 2000 to 2010 in those on ART with viral load thresholds at 50, 400, and 1000 copies/mL and found no difference in transmission according to the mode of delivery between the different cutoffs.[31] In addition, when considering delivery timing in this population, Scott and colleagues found that elective delivery before 40 weeks was not found to decrease the risk of transmission, so delivery timing should be based on standard obstetrics indications.[32]

The use of zidovudine in this population is varied with experts positing that in those receiving and compliant to ART and viral loads less than 50 copies/mL, it can be deferred. In Myer and colleagues, the risk of transmission in those on ART with viral loads of 50 to 1000 copies/mL had a 2% risk of transmission, compared 0.25% in those with viral loads less than 50 copies/mL.[33] Given concern there is a slightly increased risk of transmission in those with viral loads between 50 and 1000 copies/mL, some experts recommend intrapartum zidovudine despite a viral load less than 1000 copies/mL. The use of intrapartum zidovudine should be individualized based on antiretroviral compliance, in discussion with the patient considering their preferences.

Other Intrapartum Considerations

There are other processes that should be followed for all patients with HIV in labor, regardless of viral load or zidovudine prophylaxis. These include:

- Avoiding fetal scalp electrodes or internal fetal monitors as much as possible
- Continuing ART throughout labor
- Avoiding the use of methergine or other ergotamines in patients taking protease inhibitors or cobicistat to avoid excessive vasoconstriction
- Avoid operative vaginal delivery if possible, particularly if viral load is greater than 50 copies/mL
- Avoid artificial rupture of membranes if possible, particularly if viral load is greater than 50 copies/mL

Postpartum Care and Follow-Up for Patients Living with Human Immunodeficiency Virus

Based on data obtained from randomized controlled trials, regardless of CD4 count or clinical status, continuation of ART in the postpartum setting is recommended to reduce the risk of disease progression and HIV transmission.[34-36] If pregnancy-related factors, such as toxicity concerns, resulted in regimen selection in the antepartum setting that contains agents that are not preferred in nonpregnant patients, modification in the regimen may need to be made after delivery.

Given the stressors of caring for a newborn, it has been shown that adherence to ART is especially challenging in the postpartum setting,[37] which underscores the importance of adherence counseling and ensuring appropriate support before discharge from the hospital.

Breastfeeding Recommendations

Breastfeeding is not recommended in the United States or any resource-rich countries.[38] In the antepartum setting, patients should be counseled as such, even in cases of complete adherence to ART and objective evidence of viral suppression. This recommendation is based on trials in resource-limited settings demonstrating that although ART and viral suppression significantly reduce the risk of HIV transmission, they do not completely eliminate it.[39] Given the accessibility, affordability, and safety of infant formula in the United States, the risk of viral transmission with breastfeeding outweighs the known benefits of breastfeeding and is therefore not recommended. Patients should be counseled about means of lactation suppression, including wearing tight-fitting sports bras, hot and cold compresses, and pain relief from ibuprofen or acetaminophen.

Patients may, however, decide to breastfeed for a whole host of social, cultural, and personal reasons. For patients who choose to breastfeed despite the CDC recommendations, providers should counsel patients about measures to help prevent viral transmission, including continuation of ART and infant prophylaxis.[40] All infants born to mothers with HIV should receive 4 to 6 weeks of postexposure prophylaxis. Whether this duration should be extended in breastfed infants depends on maternal viral load and ART adherence. In mothers with an undetectable viral load and consistent adherence to ART, there does not seem to be a benefit to continuing infant prophylaxis for the duration of breastfeeding.[41] However, for infants of mothers who are not virally suppressed, daily prophylaxis with nevirapine until at least 1 week after weaning is recommended, as it has been shown to prevent viral transmission.[41] Regardless of the regimen and the duration of prophylaxis, it is recommended that breastfed infants should be monitored for HIV acquisition every 3 months during breastfeeding and 4 to 6 weeks, 3 months, and 6 months following the cessation of breastfeeding.

Neonatal Management

It is recommended that all infants at high risk of vertical transmission receive combination antiretroviral postexposure prophylaxis. Those who were diagnosed with acute or primary HIV during pregnancy or lactation, did not receive ART during pregnancy, those who received only intrapartum ART, or received ART, but did not achieve viral suppression (defined as HIV viral ribonucleic acid [RNA] levels of < 50 copies/mL) at least 4 weeks before delivery are considered at high risk of vertical transmission. The recommended regimen is effectively presumptive HIV treatment and includes a 6-week course of three drugs: zidovudine, lamivudine, and either treatment dose nevirapine or raltegravir. If there is concern for HIV-2, the raltegravir regimen should be used as nevirapine is ineffective against HIV-2. If zidovudine toxicity develops, abacavir can be used as an alternative. Of note, if the infant is diagnosed with HIV infection, this regimen should be continued indefinitely.

In contrast, it is recommended that infants at low risk of vertical HIV acquisition (mothers who are adherent to ART and achieve viral suppression at least 4 weeks before delivery) receive a single-drug regimen of zidovudine postexposure prophylaxis after birth for 4 to 6 weeks. All postexposure prophylaxis regimens should be initiated as soon as possible, within 6 to 12 hours of birth.

Postpartum Contraception

Patients living with HIV should be counseled regarding contraception options in light of potential drug–drug interactions between certain methods and antiretroviral drugs that may reduce the efficacy of the contraceptive method, the antiretroviral drug, or both. We recommend consulting with a pharmacist familiar with antiretroviral medications before prescribing oral contraceptive pills, using injectable contraception, or using progesterone-releasing implants.

Further Resources

For those with remaining questions or for advice about specific scenarios, the National Perinatal HIV Hotline (1–888–448–8765) provides free consultations to anyone caring for pregnant patients with HIV. Clinicians can also reference the "Recommendations for the Use of Antiretroviral Drugs During Pregnancy and Interventions to Reduce Perinatal HIV Transmission in the United States" from the US Department of Health and Human Services, available online and updated regularly.[42] Finally, clinicians can consult the National Clinician Consultation Center at the University of California San Francisco: https://nccc.ucsf.edu. Finally, the Society for Maternal-Fetal Medicine has checklists available to ensure complete care for patients living with HIV.[43]

SUMMARY

All pregnant people should be offered opt-out HIV testing at least once during pregnancy. Treatment with ART, as well as intrapartum measures and neonatal prophylaxis, can reduce the risk of perinatal HIV transmission to less than 1%.

CLINICS CARE POINTS

- All pregnant patients should be offered opt-out human immunodeficiency virus (HIV) testing during pregnancy.
- Patients of reproductive age living with HIV should be asked about their reproductive intentions.
- Patients living with HIV who have serodiscordant partners should be counseled about the use of pre-exposure prophylaxis in the setting of attempting conception.
- All patients, including those who are pregnant, who are living with HIV should be started on antiretroviral therapy regardless of viral load or symptoms.
- Pregnant patients with an HIV RNA viral load less than 1000 copies/mL should only have a cesarean delivery for obstetric indications.
- Pregnant patients with an HIV RNA viral load $\leq$ 1000 copies/mL should be counseled that a prelabor/pre-rupture of membranes should be counseled that a cesarean may reduce the risk of perinatal transmission.

- Intravenous zidovudine prophylaxis at the time of delivery will help reduce the risk of perinatal transmission for most patients.
- Patients living with HIV in high-resource settings should be counseled about the Centers for Disease Control and Prevention recommendation to avoid breastfeeding.
- Neonatal prophylaxis with antiretroviral therapy will help reduce perinatal transmission.
- Multiple hotlines and clinical resources exist to help tailor recommendations to specific clinical scenarios.

CONFLICT OF INTEREST

The author reports no conflicts of interest.

REFERENCES

1. Centers for Disease Control and Prevention. Estimated HIV incidence and prevalence in the United States, 2015 - 2019. HIV surveillance supplemental report 2021; 26(No. 1). 2021. Available at: http://www.cdc.gov/hiv/library/reports/hiv-surveillance.html. Accessed November 15, 2022.
2. Nesheim SR, FitzHarris LF, Lampe MA, et al. Reconsidering the number of women with HIV infection who give birth annually in the United States. Public Health Rep 2018;133(6):637–43.
3. Connor EM, Sperling RS, Gelber R, et al. Reduction of maternal-infant transmission of human immunodeficiency virus type 1 with zidovudine treatment. Pediatric AIDS Clinical Trials Group Protocol 076 Study Group. N Engl J Med 1994;331(18): 1173–80.
4. Dorenbaum A, Cunningham CK, Gelber RD, et al. Two-dose intrapartum/newborn nevirapine and standard antiretroviral therapy to reduce perinatal HIV transmission: a randomized trial. JAMA 2002;288(2):189–98.
5. Fowler MG, Qin M, Fiscus SA, et al. Benefits and Risks of Antiretroviral Therapy for Perinatal HIV Prevention. N Engl J Med 2016;375(18):1726–37.
6. Centers for Disease Control and Prevention. HIV surveillance report. 2018. 31. Available at: https://www.cdc.gov/hiv/library/reports/hiv-surveillance/vol-31/content/children.html. Accessed November 15, 2022.
7. Centers for Disease Control and Prevention. HIV surveillance report. 2016. 28. Available at: http://www.cdc.gov/hiv/library/reports/hiv-surveillance/html. Accessed November 15, 2022.
8. Tuomala RE, Kalish LA, Zorilla C, et al. Changes in total, CD4+, and CD8+ lymphocytes during pregnancy and 1 year postpartum in human immunodeficiency virus-infected women. The Women and Infants Transmission Study. Obstet Gynecol 1997;89(6):967–74.
9. Tang JH, Sheffield JS, Grimes J, et al. Effect of protease inhibitor therapy on glucose intolerance in pregnancy. Obstet Gynecol 2006;107(5):1115–9.
10. Lathrop E, Jamieson DJ, Danel I. HIV and maternal mortality. Int J Gynaecol Obstet 2014;127(2):213–5.
11. Wedi CO, Kirtley S, Hopewell S, et al. Perinatal outcomes associated with maternal HIV infection: a systematic review and meta-analysis. Lancet HIV 2016;3(1):e33–48.
12. Pollock L, Cohan D, Pecci CC, et al, ACOG Committee Opinion No. 752. Prenatal and perinatal human immunodeficiency virus testing. Obstet Gynecol 2019; 133(1):187.

13. US Preventative Services Task Force, Owens DK, Davidson KW, Krist AH, et al. Screening for HIV Infection: US Preventive Services Task Force Recommendation Statement. JAMA 2019;321(23):2326–36.

14. Branson BM, Handsfield HH, Lampe MA, et al. Revised recommendations for HIV testing of adults, adolescents, and pregnant women in health-care settings. MMWR Recomm Rep 2006;55(RR-14):1–17.

15. Centers for Disease Control and Prevention. HIV testing among pregnant women–United States and Canada, 1998-2001. MMWR Morb Mortal Wkly Rep 2002;51(45):1013–6.

16. Cassimatis IR, Ayala LD, Miller ES, et al. Third-trimester repeat HIV testing: it is time we make it universal. Am J Obstet Gynecol 2021;225(5):494–9.

17. Nasrullah M, Wesolowski LG, Meyer WA 3rd, et al. Performance of a fourth-generation HIV screening assay and an alternative HIV diagnostic testing algorithm. AIDS 2013;27(5):731–7.

18. National Center for HIV/AIDS VH, and TB Prevention (U.S.). Division of HIV/AIDS Prevention, Association of Public Health Laboratories. Quick reference guide: recommended laboratory HIV testing algorithm for serum or plasma specimens. 2018. Centers for Disease Control and Prevention, Atlanta, GA.

19. Eisinger RW, Dieffenbach CW, Fauci AS. HIV viral load and transmissibility of HIV infection: undetectable equals untransmittable. JAMA 2019;321(5):451–2.

20. Centers for Disease Control and Prevention. HIV Treatment as Prevention. Available at: https://www.cdc.gov/hiv/risk/art/index.html. Accessed November 15, 2022.

21. Centers for Disease Control and Prevention. Available at: https://www.cdc.gov/vaccines/adults/rec-vac/health-conditions/hiv.html. Accessed November 15, 2022.

22. Floridia M, Masuelli G, Meloni A, et al. Amniocentesis and chorionic villus sampling in HIV-infected pregnant women: a multicentre case series. BJOG 2017;124(8):1218–23.

23. Wang L, Kourtis AP, Ellington S, et al. Safety of tenofovir during pregnancy for the mother and fetus: a systematic review. Clin Infect Dis 2013;57(12):1773–81.

24. Rasi V, Cortina-Borja M, Peters H, et al. Brief Report: surveillance of congenital anomalies after exposure to raltegravir or elvitegravir during pregnancy in the United Kingdom and Ireland, 2008-2018. J Acquir Immune Defic Syndr 2019;80(3):264–8.

25. Floridia M, Mastroiacovo P, Tamburrini E, et al. Birth defects in a national cohort of pregnant women with HIV infection in Italy, 2001-2011. BJOG 2013;120(12):1466–75.

26. European Mode of Delivery Collaboration. Elective caesarean-section versus vaginal delivery in prevention of vertical HIV-1 transmission: a randomised clinical trial. Lancet 1999;353(9158):1035–9.

27. ACOG Committee Opinion No. 751 Summary: labor and delivery management of women with human immunodeficiency virus infection. Obstet Gynecol 2018;132(3):803–4.

28. Minkoff H, Burns DN, Landesman S, et al. The relationship of the duration of ruptured membranes to vertical transmission of human immunodeficiency virus. Am J Obstet Gynecol 1995;173(2):585–9.

29. International Perinatal HIV Group. Duration of ruptured membranes and vertical transmission of HIV-1: a meta-analysis from 15 prospective cohort studies. AIDS 2001;15(3):357–68.

30. Townsend CL, Cortina-Borja M, Peckham CS, et al. Low rates of mother-to-child transmission of HIV following effective pregnancy interventions in the United Kingdom and Ireland, 2000-2006. AIDS 2008;22(8):973–81.
31. Briand N, Jasseron C, Sibiude J, et al. Cesarean section for HIV-infected women in the combination antiretroviral therapies era, 2000-2010. Am J Obstet Gynecol 2013;209(4):335 e331–e335 e312.
32. Scott RK, Chakhtoura N, Burke MM, et al. Delivery after 40 weeks of gestation in pregnant women with well-controlled human immunodeficiency virus. Obstet Gynecol 2017;130(3):502–10.
33. Myer L, Phillips TK, McIntyre JA, et al. HIV viraemia and mother-to-child transmission risk after antiretroviral therapy initiation in pregnancy in Cape Town, South Africa. HIV Med 2017;18(2):80–8.
34. Group ISS, Lundgren JD, Babiker AG, et al. Initiation of antiretroviral therapy in early asymptomatic HIV infection. N Engl J Med 2015;373(9):795–807.
35. Cohen MS, Chen YQ, McCauley M, et al. Prevention of HIV-1 infection with early antiretroviral therapy. N Engl J Med 2011;365(6):493–505.
36. Grinsztejn B, Hosseinipour MC, Ribaudo HJ, et al. Effects of early versus delayed initiation of antiretroviral treatment on clinical outcomes of HIV-1 infection: results from the phase 3 HPTN 052 randomised controlled trial. Lancet Infect Dis 2014; 14(4):281–90.
37. Nachega JB, Uthman OA, Anderson J, et al. Adherence to antiretroviral therapy during and after pregnancy in low-income, middle-income, and high-income countries: a systematic review and meta-analysis. AIDS 2012;26(16):2039–52.
38. Centers for Disease Control and Prevention. HIV and perinatal transmission: preventing perinatal HIV transmission. Available at: https://www.cdc.gov/hiv/group/pregnant-people/transmission.html. Accessed November 15, 2022.
39. Flynn PM, Taha TE, Cababasay M, et al. Association of maternal viral load and CD4 count with perinatal HIV-1 transmission risk during breastfeeding in the PROMISE postpartum component. J Acquir Immune Defic Syndr 2021;88(2): 206–13.
40. Levison J, Weber S, Cohan D. Breastfeeding and HIV-infected women in the United States: harm reduction counseling strategies. Clin Infect Dis 2014;59(2): 304–9.
41. Coovadia HM, Brown ER, Fowler MG, et al. Efficacy and safety of an extended nevirapine regimen in infant children of breastfeeding mothers with HIV-1 infection for prevention of postnatal HIV-1 transmission (HPTN 046): a randomised, double-blind, placebo-controlled trial. Lancet 2012;379(9812):221–8.
42. Panel on Treatment of HIV During Pregnancy and Prevention of Perinatal Transmission. Recommendations for the use of antirertoviral drugs during pregnancy and interventions to reduce perinatal HIV transmission in the United States. Department of Health and Human Services. Available at: https://clinicalinfo.hiv.gov/en/guidelines/perinatal. Accessed November 15, 2022.
43. Patient Safety and Quality Committee, Society for Maternal-Fetal Medicine, Gibson KS, Toner LE. Society for Maternal-Fetal Medicine Special Statement: Updated checklists for pregnancy management in persons with HIV. Am J Obstet Gynecol 2020;223(5):B6–11.

Vaccine Hesitancy in Women's Health

Benjamin Spires, MD, Major, USAF, MC[a], Annabeth Brewton, MD[b], Jill M. Maples, PhD[b], Samantha F. Ehrlich, PhD, MPH[c], Kimberly B. Fortner, MD[b],*

KEYWORDS

- Vaccine • Vaccine hesitancy • Maternal immunization • Delayed vaccination
- COVID vaccine in pregnancy

KEY POINTS

- Vaccine hesitancy has been defined as: a delay in acceptance of vaccination; a refusal of vaccination despite availability of the vaccine; or a state of indecision and uncertainty about vaccination.
- Vaccine hesitancy poses a significant threat to public health with direct impact to several vaccines that important to women's health and their providers.
- Technology and internet-based platforms (ie, social media) are convenient sources of health-related materials and education; however have contributed to detrimental dispersion of vaccine misinformation.
- Identification and understanding of specific concerns or challenges in the hesitancy continuum may help public health and individual medical providers are essential in the journey to impact vaccine uptake.

INTRODUCTION

Since their discovery, vaccines have been considered one of the top ten achievements in public health during the 20th Century.[1,2] Vaccines reduce morbidity and mortality from the disease they are preventing and improve the health and lifespan of an individual and population in which they live.[3] Following the coordination of vaccine administration into national and international immunization programs, many diseases impacting childhood survival have been reduced (neonatal tetanus) and a few eradicated (naturally occurring smallpox).[4] Further, the World Health Organization

[a] Department of Ob/Gyn, Uniformed Services University of the Health Sciences, 307 Boatner Road, Eglin Air Force Base, FL 32542, USA; [b] Department of Ob/Gyn, University of Tennessee Graduate School of Medicine, 1924 Alcoa Highway, Box U-27, Knoxville, TN 37920, USA; [c] Department of Public Health, University of Tennessee, 369 HPER, 1914 Andy Holt Avenue, Knoxville, TN 37996, USA
* Corresponding author. Office of Women and Infants Center of Excellence, University of Tennessee Medical Center, 1924 Alcoa Highway, Box 96, Knoxville, TN 37920.
E-mail address: kfortner@utmck.edu

Obstet Gynecol Clin N Am 50 (2023) 401–419
https://doi.org/10.1016/j.ogc.2023.02.013
0889-8545/23/© 2023 Elsevier Inc. All rights reserved.

obgyn.theclinics.com

estimates that over 3,000,000 deaths are prevented each year by immunization programs.[3] Millions of healthcare dollars are conserved based on mitigation of vaccine preventable disease, through cost per case prevented, cost per life saved, cost per life-year saved, and cost per quality-adjusted life year saved (QALY).[5] Specifically, in a meta-analysis examining cost effectiveness of adult vaccination, influenza and pneumococcal vaccination are estimated to have a cost effectiveness ratio of < $50,000 per QALY saved while HPV vaccination has a cost effectiveness ratio of < $100,000 per QALY.[5] While many providers and patients consider vaccines an improvement in healthcare, there are persistently individuals who decline all vaccines, a vaccine, or a specific schedule of vaccination. Vaccine hesitancy has been defined as: a delay in acceptance of vaccination; a refusal of vaccination despite availability of the vaccine; or a state of indecision and uncertainty about vaccination.[6] The World Health Organization describes vaccine hesitancy as patient-level reluctance to receive vaccines.[7] Vaccination sources agree that hesitancy varies by time, place, particular vaccine, and is influenced by vaccine availability, affordability, and accessibility.[8] Cultural and social influences also play a part in the decision to be vaccinated; however, individual determinants of hesitancy are the aspect that providers are more likely to impact in a clinical encounter.[9] This review will focus on some of the basics of vaccine components, definitions of vaccine hesitancy, review specific examples of vaccines administered in women's health, and consequences of vaccine refusal, as well as potential strategies to reduce or minimize hesitancy among our patients.

Vaccine Basics

In order to understand more about vaccine hesitancy, a general review of vaccine principles, platforms, and components is essential. Vaccines are designed to introduce a nonthreatening portion of virus or bacteria to our immune system and thereby elicit a response from both B-cell (humoral immune responses), and T-cell (cell-mediated) immune responses. Antigenic components range from whole cell pertussis to purified proteins to toxoids (like diphtheria) to the manufacturing of a spike protein (as in COVID).

Vaccine platforms are widely varied and refer to the type of antigenic target that each vaccine system uses. At this point in time, there are at least 7 types of vaccine platforms which are listed below.[4] Antigenic targets include.

1. Live or attenuated bacteria or virus capable of inducing immunity can be used in an immune-competent recipient without causing illness, much like the oral polio vaccine or MMR vaccine.[10]
2. Killed whole organism, rendered non-infectious by heat or other sources, can then be used even in immunodeficient recipients to generate immunity, with an example being the whole cell pertussis vaccine (DTP), or rabies.[11]
3. Toxoids (or toxins produced by bacteria) can be the basis for a vaccine when present in trace and inactivated forms as in the case of tetanus or diphtheria.
4. A subunit or portion of a purified protein, recombinant protein, peptide or polysaccharide can be administered in a vaccine. Examples of this include the pertussis components of Tdap,[10] pneumococcal, and some of the candidate GBS vaccines.
5. Virus-like particles consist of small portions of the virus or nanopeptide/protein(s) that lack viral genome and are placed onto another protein often with inclusion of an adjuvant to boost the immune response, for example, HPV vaccine.[12]
6. Viral vectored vaccines where the pathogen is engineered or incorporated into a benign or attenuated strain of a different virus. Examples of this type of vaccine

include the 2019 Ebola vaccine, and Janssen/Johnson & Johnson COVID-vaccine.[13]
7. Nucleic acid vaccines contain a small portion of messenger RNA that is stabilized and used to inject into the recipient, and then the recipient's cellular machinery makes a copy of the protein which then induces an immune response. Examples include the Pfizer[14] and Moderna[15] COVID vaccines.

Vaccine components refer to everything in-between that allows the vaccine platform to be injected and effective. Vaccines often contain small amounts of preservatives, stabilizers, residuals, surfactant, and adjuvants.[4] Preservatives are usually present in small amounts and keep the vaccine stable for storage and distribution. Stabilizers may include gelatin or sorbitol. Residuals are trace amounts of the substances utilized in the manufacturing process which carries over to the final distributed vaccine product (eg, stabilizers, egg proteins). Residuals usually exist in such small quantities ('trace amounts') that no known health risks have been demonstrated. Some of the hesitancy movement focuses on the residuals (particularly preservatives) despite lack of supporting evidence. Adjuvants are used to improve or boost the recipient's immune response, often with inactivated vaccines. Common adjuvants include aluminum sulfate (alum)[16] which is in some Hepatitis B and pneumococcal vaccines and MF59,[17] and oil in water emulsion, which is included in some influenza vaccines.

Vaccine Hesitancy

Vaccine hesitancy can lead individuals to delay or adjust recommended vaccine schedules, partially vaccinate, or decline vaccination altogether.[8,18–20] Less than ideal vaccination rates were noted prior to the pandemic to the extent that the World Health Organization (WHO) identified hesitancy to vaccines as one of the Top Ten Threats to Global Health in 2019.[20] Vaccine hesitancy was preceded on WHO's list only by the concern for global influenza pandemic, Ebola, and other high-threat pathogens. Decades before the COVID-19 pandemic, evidence of increasing vaccine hesitancy was emerging. In particular, increasing numbers of parents were declining or delaying their children's recommended vaccinations, citing frustration with school or government vaccine requirements/schedules, lack of trust in vaccines, and the report of negative health outcomes synchronous with vaccine receipt.[21] Unfortunately, the COVID pandemic seems to have heightened existing hesitancy sentiments, expanding the impact from decisions adults make for their children to decisions they also make for themselves.

Characterizing predictors of vaccine hesitancy are challenging. Different public health authorities and working groups have attempted to understand the most important systematic and patient-level factors, behaviors, and beliefs that result in vaccine hesitancy. The Aspen Institute's Sabin Vaccine group published their 2020 report posing that hesitancy may originate from: (1) restrictions, such as inconvenience in accessing vaccines, both individually and system level with intermittent supply shortages, (2) affordability of vaccines, (3) lessened confidence in their efficacy, and (4) diminished concerns over disease/illnesses they prevent. Among all barriers identified, a consistent challenge centers around misinformation. Vaccine misinformation ranges from concerns about the health benefits of vaccine or impact of disease, the vaccine composition, to the adverse events following immunization (AEFI). According to a 2021 Kaiser survey regarding COVID-19 vaccines, vaccine hesitancy also seems to be a continuum of beliefs and behaviors around whether or not to accept vaccination, representing more of a spectrum from cautious acceptors to outright deniers with individuals seeking more information or access making up the "moveable middle."[22] It is important to recognize and understand the differences in level of hesitancy to direct appropriate energy and effect change.

Prior to the COVID-19 pandemic, WHO designated the Strategic Advisory Group of Experts on Immunization (SAGE) and their work defined the components of hesitancy as: complacency, confidence, and convenience.[8,23,24] Complacency refers to the perception that the risks of vaccine-preventable diseases remain low. Confidence refers to trust in the safety and effectiveness of vaccines, the health care system, and policymakers who recommend vaccines. Convenience refers to the availability, affordability, and accessibility of vaccines, meaning ease of access to receiving vaccine. Additional groups have added two more "C"s, asserting the importance of Compassion and Collective, referring to collective action, collective responsibility to public health, and health authorities using a more collective identity.[24,25] See **Fig. 1**.

Technology and internet-based tools are convenient resources for obtaining health-related educational materials and information. Medically accurate vaccine information also appears widely across social media platforms.[26] Social media allows individuals and communities to communicate and share information, personal opinions, and other content. Individuals have increasingly relied on social media for vaccine-related information that is not always scientifically reviewed, and there are concerns about the large-scale spread of misinformation related to medical research and a strong potential for polarized views regarding vaccination to be amplified.[27] Oi-Yee Li and colleagues published in the British Medical Journal Global Health, reviewing over 150 English-speaking YouTube videos that were related to COVID-19 or coronavirus. Nearly one-fourth of the YouTube videos contained non-factual information or were misleading, despite having already accumulated over 62 million views while videos from reputable sources were vastly underrepresented.[28]

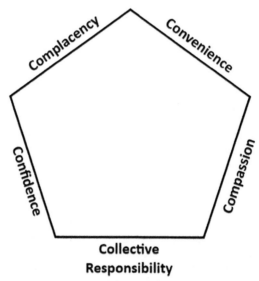

Fig. 1. Intersection of factors contributing to vaccine hesitancy. (*Adapted from* MacDonald NE; SAGE Working Group on Vaccine Hesitancy. Vaccine hesitancy: Definition, scope and determinants and Battarbee AN, et al. Attitudes Toward COVID-19 Illness and COVID-19 Vaccination among Pregnant Women: A Cross-Sectional Multicenter Study during August-December 2020; with permission.)

Irrespective of social media platform, spreading patterns and content sharing persist regardless of the accuracy of the information. Social media reaches larger audiences simply by "liking", following, or retweeting.[29] At the height of the COVID-19 pandemic, every 45 milliseconds, there was a tweet containing #coronavirus, and retweeting was notably higher with antivaccine sentiments.[29] Blankenship at all compared two vaccine-related Twitter datasets and found that any tweet containing antivaccine sentiments (often marked with #vaxxed #CDCwhistleblower) was 4.13 times more likely to be retweeted; while pro-vaccine tweets were retweeted 1.58 times when compared to neutral vaccine tweets.[30,31] Additionally, user selection does not even begin to combat the power of content-polluting bots that can outpace any human tweeting activity.[32]

The impact of social media on vaccine opposition was identified before the COVID-19 pandemic; however, the COVID-19 pandemic amplified how social media may have increased vaccine hesitancy. In March of 2019, the CEO of the American Medical Association published a letter urging social media companies to better promote or ensure accurate information on the safety and efficacy of vaccines on their social media platforms.[33] Measures to control the COVID-19 pandemic potentially heightened the impact from social media, specifically: (1) social isolation and physical distancing was one of the strategies implemented to control the pandemic, which led to (2) many remaining in isolation with intensified use of social media. (3) As social media users engaged in social media content selection with "thumbs up" or "thumbs down", (4) these selection decisions further invested users in platform algorithms and resulted in (5) aggregation of users into clusters. These clusters are ideologic sub-communities commonly known as "Echo chambers". Vaccine hesitancy content in social media creates many challenges whether people or robot driven selections are made, social media platforms are able to provide unconfirmed information that out reaches, outpaces, and over influences standard/traditional media or public health officials and their website content.[28]

Specific Vaccine Examples

Human papillomavirus (HPV) vaccine

HPV is a sexually transmitted double-stranded deoxyribonucleic acid (DNA) virus that can lead to oropharyngeal and anogenital cancers, most notably, cervical cancer. HPV vaccines which provide protection from certain high-risk HPV types associated with cancer have been approved for use in the United States since 2006. The Advisory Committee on Immunization Practices (ACIP) and American College of Obstetricians and Gynecologists (ACOG) currently recommend routine HPV vaccination for children ages 11 to 12 but vaccination is also approved for use in both males and females from ages 9 to 45.[34,35] When given prior to initial HPV exposure, the vaccine is highly effective at preventing infection against the more virulent HPV subtypes as evidenced by declining HPV infection following the U.S. HPV vaccination program.[36] Despite demonstrated efficacy, vaccine hesitancy remains high as demonstrated by lower vaccine uptake when compared to other recommended ACIP vaccines. The CDC's TeenVaxView reports that approximately 76% of U.S. adolescents (both males and females) aged 13 to 17 have received one dose of the HPV vaccine as of 2021. Only 49% to 57% have completed the HPV vaccine series. This is compared to 89% to 92% receiving Tdap and 85% to 89% receiving quadrivalent meningococcal conjugate vaccine.[37]

Because HPV vaccine is ideally given to adolescents, vaccine hesitancy starts with parents, or guardians, affecting younger OB/Gyn patients and older pediatric patients. A 2020 report by Szilagy and colleagues, surveyed families of adolescents across the

U.S. and demonstrated that nearly one-fourth of parents (23% of 2020 respondents) were hesitant about the HPV vaccine. Adolescents of these hesitant parents were a third less likely to have received at least one dose of the vaccine (21% vs 74% of 2020 respondents).[38] Common concerns from parents regarding the HPV vaccine included: efficacy, safety, the relatively recent production and approval of the vaccine, and lack of belief that the vaccine benefits their teen. Tsui and colleagues conducted in-depth interviews among multi-specialty providers (family medicine and pediatric) in New Jersey during the summer of 2019, and every provider reported encountering some level of hesitancy from parents when introducing the HPV vaccine. Their data revealed that vaccine hesitancy reasons included: misinformation and mistrust expressed by parents; increased time requirements/interruptions in physician work-flow to offer vaccine education; and inconsistencies within the health system when HPV vaccine is recommended by the teenage provider but omitted from middle school vaccine requirements. In addition to patient-level and systems-based hesitancy, re-gion of care also appears to have a unique impact on HPV vaccine hesitancy. In 2019, Williams and colleagues used data from the National Immunization Survey and found that teens living in suburban or rural areas were more hesitant to receive HPV vaccine as well as residence in the Southern United States.[39] Reasons for geographic differences in hesitancy remain unclear and data are compounded by con-sistency of keeping the age 11 to 12 well-child visit.[39]

Additional apprehension from parents regarding adolescent HPV vaccination is the misconception of increased promiscuity among those who have received the vaccine. There is no evidence of riskier sexual behavior or higher rates of sexually transmitted diseases among vaccinated individuals. In fact, vaccinated individuals were found to have lower rates of Chlamydia and higher rates of condom and other contraception use.[40]

HPV vaccine misinformation and lack of provider recommendation also contribute to less-than-ideal HPV vaccine uptake. Patients considering HPV vaccination may find a host of concerns on social media including alleged risk for autoimmune disor-ders, neurologic conditions, venous thrombotic events, and infertility. None of these concerns have been demonstrated in either prelicensure or post-licensure reported literature, yet this misinformation contributes to vaccine hesitancy.[41–43] HPV vaccine hesitancy is not only a problem with patients, but also the healthcare providers recom-mending these vaccines. McRee et al found that only 76% of providers included in the study would routinely recommend the HPV vaccine to adolescent girls and only 46% to adolescent boys. About half of these providers felt they did not have enough time to discuss the parents' concerns or felt as if they would be unable to change their par-ents' minds anyway. This study demonstrates that even perhaps perceived patient hesitancy by clinicians could also affect vaccination rates.[44]

Seasonal Influenza Vaccine

Influenza vaccine has had longstanding resistance among the general population, pregnant and nonpregnant persons. The impact of poor vaccine uptake is heightened among pregnant persons given increased risks of influenza illness. For those reasons, the focus of influenza vaccine hesitancy discussed here will be through the context of pregnancy, recognizing many of the concerns and limitations can be applied to nonpregnant populations.

Seasonal influenza vaccine should be offered annually to all pregnant persons, regardless of trimester of pregnancy starting in September or October and continuing through the end of flu season, generally May/June.[45,46] Pregnant people have demon-strated hesitancy to accept seasonal influenza vaccination for decades and Women's

Health Providers have had first-hand experience. Uptake rates of seasonal influenza vaccine were as low as 13% to 24% prior to H1N1 pandemic influenza season increasing to 41% in areas following H1N1, during 2013 to 14 season.[47,48] The current century includes two prior respiratory pandemics: Influenza H1N1 Pandemic and COVID-19, both of which appear to have heightened influenza vaccine hesitancy.[49] A 2019 study from California evaluated influenza uptake along over 77,000 women by sociodemographic factors, finding lower rates of vaccine uptake among women of color, Hispanic ethnicity, and subsidized insurance. Lower uptake was also noted among women with fewer prenatal care visits suggesting convenience of vaccine administration played a role in hesitancy.[50]

Lack of confidence in influenza vaccine safety and efficacy have been contributing factors nationally and worldwide. Influenza safety concerns are broad and range from association with miscarriage,[51] maternal safety (as in medically attended allergic or local events, thrombocytopenia, and neurologic events),[52] and congenital anomalies.[53–55] Using Vaccine Safety Datalink data, large cohorts, clinical trials, and systematic reviews and meta-analyses, no safety signals have been identified for the mother, fetus, pregnancy, or early childhood.[56] While avoiding the influenza vaccine during the first trimester was initially to decrease coincident timing of vaccination and pregnancy loss, this practice may have created mixed messaging. Given seasonal nature of influenza and need to produce the new vaccine annually, many pose questions about the feasibility of testing new vaccines every year. The effectiveness of influenza vaccine during pregnancy is supported by data demonstrating reductions in adverse obstetric outcomes such as stillbirth,[57] preterm birth, and small for gestational age infants).[58,59] There are also some studies reporting neutral findings, creating an opportunity for doubt/hesitancy. Two recent meta-analyses performed in 2014 and 2018 summarized available data demonstrating less influenza-like illness among pregnant people following receipt of H1N1 containing influenza vaccines by 89% (CI 79–94) and that children born to mothers who received flu vaccination had reduced laboratory confirmed influenza (41%, 95% CI: 6–63).[60,61] Over a decade of literature has supported the effectiveness of seasonal flu vaccination in mitigating maternal illness, improving obstetric outcomes, and providing vertical transmission of antibodies for newborn protection; yet, influenza uptake rates remain low.[60–62]

Influenza vaccine hesitancy is significantly affected by complacency to illness among all populations, and pregnancy is no different. A systematic review from 2017 found decreases in perceived risks of getting the flu, complications from the flu, susceptibility to the flu, and cite lack of prior adverse events from the flu as reason for hesitancy among pregnant patients, as well as nearly all populations studied.[63] Another frequently reported patient-level concern about influenza vaccination is patient's state that they "get the flu" following vaccination, potentially based on temporal association of viral illness or malaise with vaccine receipt.[64] Internationally, a 2021 systematic review that included 11 studies from Western Europe examined influenza vaccine hesitancy among pregnant women. Key factors in hesitancy identified were: concerns about safety, risks to mother and child, the low perception of risk in the general population of becoming truly ill from influenza, and questioning the effectiveness of the vaccine.[65]

Discussion of influenza vaccine hesitancy without inclusion of thimerosal would be incomplete. Thimerosal, an antimicrobial agent used as a vaccine preservative, has long been cited as a vaccine safety controversy, with initial discussions occurring in 1990s.[66] Thimerosal contains ethyl mercury, in small amounts, rather than the more dangerous methylmercury and does not remain in the body or accumulate with consecutive vaccines resulting in harm.[42] The myths surrounding thimerosal link this vaccine preservative to increased risk for autism and neuro developmental issues. The original 1998 paper by Wakefield and colleagues initially raising concern that thimerosal could be linked to adverse neurodevelopmental issues was retracted nearly a decade later (2010).[42] A meta-analysis including over 1.2 million children examining longitudinal studies has not found any substantiating link between autism and thimerosal-containing vaccines.[67] Further, when examining data on receipt of flu vaccines containing thimerosal during pregnancy, there are no associations with adverse early childhood neurodevelopmental outcomes.[68]

Tetanus, Diphtheria, and acellular Pertussis (Tdap) vaccine

Since the introduction of vaccination against tetanus, diphtheria, and pertussis, incidence of these diseases has decreased drastically. The first tetanus toxoid-containing vaccines were introduced in the mid-1940s. Since then, the rates of reported tetanus in the US decreased by over 98%, with the annual incidence as reported by the Centers for Disease Control and Prevention (CDC) in 2016 of 0.01 per 100,0000. A comparable trend is seen in reported cases of diphtheria since the universal vaccination of children in the late 1940s from 200,000 cases in 1921 to only 13 reported cases in the US from 1996 to 2016.[69] Internationally, the World Health Organization continues work to reduce life threatening consequences of non-sterilized delivery from tetanus infection through tetanus vaccination via their Maternal and Neonatal Tetanus Elimination (MNTE) campaign with noted declines over the last two decades.[70] Unlike tetanus and diphtheria, however, cases of pertussis continue to increase. Some evidence suggests that this increase over the past four decades could be due to waning natural immunity and decreased vaccination uptake over time after the vaccine was changed to acellular pertussis in the 1990s.[69]

Due to the waning immunity of all components of the Tdap vaccine, various forms of the vaccine are recommended throughout one's lifespan. The ACIP recommends infants and children receive 5 doses of diphtheria-tetanus-acellular pertussis (DTaP) from ages 2 months to 6 years. Adolescents should then receive a single dose of Tdap at 11 to 12 years. A booster with either Tdap or tetanus toxoid and reduced diphtheria toxoid (Td) every 10 years.[71]

Because DTaP is not given to newborn infants until 2 months of age, this population experiences the greatest morbidity and mortality associated with pertussis, or whooping cough as it is commonly referred to. As a result of this, ACOG, along with the ACIP, recommend Tdap be administered to all pregnant individuals, ideally from 27 to 36 weeks gestation.[71,72] By immunizing pregnant people, maternal antibodies are then transferred across the placenta to provide protection to the infant after birth.

Multiple studies have been conducted to evaluate the safety and efficacy of Tdap during pregnancy. In a large study out of Keiser Permanente Southern California that evaluated Tdap safety during pregnancy for both mother and fetus, no increased risk was noted in either mother or infant in any of the pre-specified outcomes when Tdap was given after 27 weeks' gestation.[73] A randomized controlled trial by Munoz and colleagues evaluating maternal vaccination at 30 to 32 weeks' gestation found no increased risk of adverse events among women or their infants. The study did find high concentrations of infant pertussis antibodies during the first 2 months of life.[74] Even with these recommendations, Tdap uptake during pregnancy remains low. In a survey conducted by the CDC in 2021, only 53.5% of patients reported receiving the vaccine during pregnancy. Lack of knowledge was the most common reason for declining vaccine, with almost half of respondents stating they did not know they needed a Tdap with each pregnancy, highlighting a potential gap in patient directed public health information. Other concerns from survey participants related more to questions about safety of the vaccine for both the mother and her fetus.[75] In a survey of 325 unvaccinated pregnant women, 81% and 92% of participants believed pertussis infection would be serious or very serious for themselves or their infants, respectively. Despite this concern, only 44% stated they were likely to receive the Tdap vaccine during pregnancy.[76] Like other vaccines, when evaluating US and international data, the consistent themes around Tdap hesitancy focus on perception that risk of infection with pertussis is low, pertussis illness severity is low, concerns about the safety of the vaccination in pregnancy, and overall mistrust of the information available about the Tdap vaccine.[49,77]

COVID vaccine

By far, the newest recommended vaccine to be given during pregnancy are the COVID-19 vaccines. The American College of Obstetricians and Gynecologists (ACOG), Society for Maternal-Fetal Medicine (SMFM),[78] and Centers for Disease Control and Prevention have all endorsed vaccination for all people age 12 and older, including people who are pregnant, lactating, and trying to achieve pregnancy now or who might become pregnant in the future.[79,80] Many felt significant relief with the release of the new mRNA COVID-19 vaccines in December 2020, and discussions over prioritizing vaccine receipt,[81] vaccine lottery's, and discussions of distribution were initiated.[82] By summer 2021 administration of COVID-19 vaccines began to dramatically fall such that discarded vaccine doses rose into the millions in the United States.[83] While initial vaccine safety assessments did not include pregnant subjects, significant post FDA EUA-release data have not revealed any safety concerns in COVID-19 vaccines administered during pregnancy or lactation.[84,85] Despite anxiety about COVID illness, even as late as December 2020, most pregnant women reported being worried about getting sick with COVID (72%) yet only 41% were considering vaccination.[23] Data from a 2022 meta-analysis report that despite viral strain, pregnant people have worse outcomes with COVID-19 infection compared to nonpregnant counterparts.[86]

Using V-Safe pregnancy registry data, mRNA COVID-19 vaccines have been given peri-conception, and in all 3 trimesters with no increased and miscarriage, stillbirth, pregnancy complication, or neonatal outcome when compared to background rates.[87,88] The vaccines have been proven effective at preventing illness[89] and are without evidence of harm.[90] Despite affirming the risks of COVID-19 infection and reassuring data on the vaccine, COVID-19 vaccine uptake remains low in pregnant women.[23,24] After vaccines were available, regardless of circulating COVID strain, vaccination uptake rates in pregnancy have hovered around 30%.[23,91]

COVID-19 vaccine hesitancy in pregnant people and of child-bearing age, has had several focuses since vaccines were released for use. Concerns have been raised regarding COVID-19 vaccines and fertility,[92,93] risk for VTE,[94] and risks to the newborn[95,96] and no significant safety signals related to these concerns have been found.[97] Early in the pandemic, social media posts contained messages of complacency - COVID-19 infection is "like a cold" or "like the flu"; "there are medicines to help me avoid intubation."[23,91] Medical sources attempted to provide accurate information in social media posts that pregnant women were "more likely to be intubated, in the ICU, on ECMO, or have death" from COVID. Confidence in COVID vaccines has also played a role in related hesitancy. From the perspective of hesitant individuals, two of the most commonly administered COVID vaccines utilized a new platform, which was then produced and distributed quickly. While precise data on vaccine research and development is not typically discussed in the non-medical community, all are generally aware that other vaccines took about a decade to arrive to full implementation and use. According to Kaiser Family Foundation poll Aug 2020, 62% affirmed belief that sociopolitical factors and pressures could lead to rushed approval to vaccine in absence of confirmed safety and efficacy, and only 42% respondents said that would be willing to receive the vaccine.[23] Confidence in health authorities was also undermined given changing or conflicting recommendations from public health authorities (the WHO recommendation that pregnant people can be vaccinated, and initially was considered if the pregnant person had increased risks compared to the CDC recommendation that vaccines not be withheld on basis of pregnancy). Exclusion of pregnant women in trials limited the initial conversations between provider and patient regarding vaccine safety in pregnancy. First-line workers receipt of vaccine and participation in real-time safety assessment systems (like CDC V-safe) aided in providing data for their pregnant peers. As Shook at al cleverly point out, the irony for clinical care providers caring for critically ill COVID- infected pregnant people that recurred with resounding measure was attempting to review risks and benefits of remdesivir, tocilizumab, or other monoclonal antibodies with far less data than the COVID vaccines that prevented or mitigated critical illness.[24] Lastly, COVID-19 vaccine receipt was also not as convenient as other vaccines given by Women's Health Providers given their unique storage requirements and varied based on people's community and state vaccine distribution plans creating barriers, perceived or real, to vaccine uptake.[24]

Consequences of Vaccine Refusal

The consequences of vaccine refusal/hesitancy impact the individual and the community as well as impacting public health. While hesitancy may reflect an individual decision, a vaccine being delayed in order to seek more information, adjust a suggested schedule, partially vaccinate, or decline the vaccine altogether also impacts their dependents and household. While individual choices should be respected, these decisions have a larger impact on herd immunity.

The concept of herd immunity is an essential aspect of epidemiology. Disease spreads by infection of susceptible hosts. As a population or "herd" accumulates immunity, either through vaccination or by prior infection, the number of susceptible hosts decreases, thereby limiting the spread of disease.[98] After a certain threshold of immunity has been reached, the immune (natural or immunized) provide protection for the unvaccinated, immunocompromised, or otherwise non-immune members by reducing susceptible hosts. An example of this was eradication of the smallpox virus after >80% of the global population was immunized.[99]

Vaccine hesitancy represents a real threat to herd immunity. Portions of the population who are hesitant about a certain vaccine can lead to vaccination rates below the threshold needed to accomplish herd immunity.[4] As an example, rates of pertussis increased over the past 4 decades, from around 4000 cases in the 1980s to over 48,000 cases in 2012. Given high transmissibility of whooping cough, around 95% of the population needs to be vaccinated to prevent outbreaks. Though overall vaccination rates worldwide remain high, rates vary significantly from 49% to 99% depending on the region and these pockets of infection contribute to further disease outbreaks.[4,100]

Another obvious example of vaccine hesitancy as a threat to herd immunity occurred with the recent COVID-19 pandemic. The WHO proposed that a vaccine coverage rate of 70% was needed for herd immunity. However, in a recent study by Plans-Rubio this number may need to be as high as 80% to 90% given transmissibility of different strains. As of April 2022, only 58.2% of the global population is fully vaccinated with 64.7% receiving at least one dose.[101] Without increased participation by the population globally, herd immunity may never be reached for COVID-19.

Potential Solutions

Interestingly, many of our patients and many of us live exclusively in silos of either vaccine acceptors or vaccine hesitancy. Social media and selective review of data can serve to confirm preconceived or fixed convictions. Lack of engaging discussion and ability to bridge the gap between these two silos has only propagated challenges in mitigating vaccine hesitancy. To quote the Sabin Aspen 2020 report, "trying to convince people with entrenched views is ineffective, and countering antivaccine narratives aggressively each time they arise may be further polarizing."[25] Perhaps there are indeed other "C"s to consider and utilize in our efforts to change vaccine hesitancy, such as collective responsibility[65] and compassion.[24]

Identification and understanding of specific concerns or challenges in the hesitancy continuum may help public health and individual medical providers in the journey to impact vaccine uptake.[102] According to a nationwide survey performed and published by the de Beaumont Foundation, some of the most important suggestions to promote vaccine acceptance may include, "tailoring your messages for specific audiences", and "explaining the benefits of getting the vaccine, not just the consequences of not taking it."[103] Higher levels of digital health literacy also appear to correlate with greater intention to vaccinate, leaving a potential opportunity to reach larger audiences.[104]

Just as healthcare providers learned that "opt out" strategies are more effective than "opt in",[105] perhaps reframing public health vaccine messages to enhance benefits may favorably impact those seeking information beyond the conversation with their health care provider. The "Fuzzy-Trace theory" is a model of cognition (memory, reasoning, and judgment) proposed by Valerie Reyna and Charles Brainard in the 1990s to predict and explain lasting memories and has been utilized to evaluate the context around healthcare decisions.[27,106] Gist or trace memories are "fuzzy" reports of a past event, representing the *bottom line* of the story rather than verbatim stories which tend to be more fact based. Gist memories appear more likely to create lasting impressions upon which personal decisions (including healthcare) are made. Further, social media posts expressing gist concepts are shared more than information offered by evidence-based medical literature.

Post Pandemic, some positive changes are happening. Discussing vaccines, their administration, and health benefits remain a focus of public health. Creating a universal influenza vaccine was mentioned in the President of the United State's 2019 Executive Order on Modernizing Influenza Vaccines in the United States to Promote Security and Public Health. Additionally, digital health literacy has changed some of the preventive healthcare landscape. At present, some social media platforms are making structural changes and partnerships to redirect vaccine posts or queries to reputable sources.[27] For example, Pinterest has redirected any vaccine related searches to a small set of hand-picked results from public health organizations including the WHO and CDC.[107] In fact, as described in the Wall Street Journal, Pinterest was the first social media to choose to banish results associated with certain vaccine-related searches regardless of whether the results might have been disreputable or reputable.[108] Facebook has also attempting to tackle vaccine misinformation by modifying algorithms to reduce ranking of antivaccine pages and rejecting advertisements with frank antivaccine messaging.[109] In the United States, Twitter has partnered with the Department of Health and Human Services to link vaccine associated keywords to vaccines.gov.[27,110] Finally in combating misinformation, platforms like

YouTube are working with high-profile content producers to widely disseminate videos and support on ways to minimize COVID-19spread.[27,111] Using narratives and leveraging celebrities appears to be at least a marginally effective method to minimize the impact of antivaccine content on social media. Often these individuals are elite users and have the greatest following, which can yield significant impact on more "viral" Tweets. Perhaps when healthcare providers personally engage in a social media platform, using anecdotal stories, imagery, and emotive language to the extent possible may have more impact.

During the COVID-19 pandemic, real-time availability to discover and convey information resulted in communities asking more questions about the safety of vaccines than previous, which can be both beneficial and challenging. The difficulty of COVID vaccine hesitancy is that it appears to impact other vaccines.[49] Multiple authors offer reminders about avoidance of judgmental language when discussing vaccine concerns or skepticism.[24,104] Further, ACOG's Committee on Ethics published their Committee Opinion on "Refusal of Medically Recommended Treatment During Pregnancy" advocating several processes to engage patients while supporting their autonomy.[112] Perhaps the 4th suggested "C" proposed by Shook and colleagues, "Compassion," should be employed in patient-provider interactions where dynamic tension exists between patient autonomy and health and wellness recommendations. Many pregnant people who refused COVID-19 vaccination did so believing they were doing the best thing for the health and wellness of their pregnancy. In addition to acknowledging this protective instinct, women's health providers will continue to readily share available data from ACOG, SMFM and CDC regarding vaccine safety. Regardless of the scientific advances in vaccine platform design, mitigating vaccine hesitancy will be necessary to prevent or minimize future vaccine preventable illness pandemics, maintain herd immunity and protect our populations, and ensure the adoption of novel vaccines.113 We must remember what Dr. George C. Benjamin, Executive Director of the American Public Hhealth Association said, "there is no one size fits all approach when it comes to vaccine communication."

DISCLOSURE

Kim Fortner serves on a Pfizer Candidate Vaccine Clinical Trial Data Safety Monitoring Committee, NCT04424316.The remaining authors have no disclosures to report.

CLINICS CARE POINTS

- The real-time release of medical information during the COVID-19 Pandemic and widespread engagement with digital media changed the way many people make healthcare decisions and connect with their healthcare providers.
- Four of the common vaccines administered by womens health providers are impacted by population-level and individual-level resistance.
- Patients and parents are hesitant regarding HPV-vaccines; however, data support the positive impact from provider recommendation and time spent to review vaccine-related concerns.
- The vaccines recommended in pregnancy, Seasonal Influenza, Tdap, and COVID, have not been associated adverse pregnancy outcomes and data suggest uptake may be aided by shared positive stories and mitigating the spread of mis-information on a personal level and among social media platforms.

REFERENCES

1. Centers for Disease Control and Prevention. Ten great public health achievements–United States, 1900-1999. MMWR Morb Mortal Wkly Rep 1999;48(12): 241–3.
2. Centers for Disease Control and Prevention. Ten great public health achievements–United States, 2001-2010. MMWR Morb Mortal Wkly Rep 2011;60(19): 619–23.
3. World Health Organization. Vaccines and immunization. WHO. Available at: https://www.who.int/health-topics/vaccines-and-immunization#tab=tab_1. Published 2022. Accessed November 14, 2022.
4. Pollard AJ, Bijker EM. A guide to vaccinology: from basic principles to new developments. Nat Rev Immunol 2021;21(2):83–100.
5. Leidner AJ, Murthy N, Chesson HW, et al. Cost-effectiveness of adult vaccinations: A systematic review. Vaccine 2019;37(2):226–34.
6. Larson HJ, Gakidou E, Murray CJL. The Vaccine-Hesitant Moment. N Engl J Med 2022;387(1):58–65.
7. World Health Organization. Vaccine hesitancy: A growing challenge for immunization programmes. WHO. Available at: https://www.who.int/news/item/18-08-2015-vaccine-hesitancy-a-growing-challenge-for-immunization-programmes. Published 2015. Accessed November 14, 2022.
8. MacDonald NE, SAGE Working Group on Vaccine Hesitancy. Vaccine hesitancy: Definition, scope and determinants. Vaccine 2015;33(34):4161–4.
9. Andersen RM. National health surveys and the behavioral model of health services use. Med Care 2008;46(7):647–53.
10. U.S. Food and Drug Administration. Measles. Mumps and Rubella Virus Vaccine Live. FDA. Available at: https://www.fda.gov/vaccines-blood-biologics/vaccines/measles-mumps-and-rubella-virus-vaccine-live. Published 2020. Accessed November 26, 2022.
11. Centers for Disease Control and Prevention. DTaP (Diphtheria, Tetanus, Pertussis) VIS. CDC. Available at: https://www.cdc.gov/vaccines/hcp/vis/vis-statements/dtap.pdf. Published 2021. Accessed November 26, 2022.
12. Merck Sharp & Dohme Corp. Gardasil (human papillomavirus quadrivalent (types 6, 11, 16, and 18) vaccine, recombinant) [package insert]. U.S. Food and Drug Administration Website. https://www.fda.gov/files/vaccines,%20blood%20&%20biologics/published/Package-Insert—Gardasil.pdf. Revised April 2015. Accessed November 26, 2022. Accessed.
13. U.S. Food and Drug Administration. Janssen. COVID-19 Vaccine. FDA. Available at: https://www.fda.gov/emergency-preparedness-and-response/coronavirus-disease-2019-covid-19/janssen-covid-19-vaccine. Published 2022. Accessed November 26, 2022.
14. U.S. Food and Drug Administration. Pfizer-BioNTech COVID-19 Vaccines. FDA. Available at: https://www.fda.gov/emergency-preparedness-and-response/coronavirus-disease-2019-covid-19/pfizer-biontech-covid-19-vaccines. Published 2022. Accessed November 26, 2022.
15. U.S. Food and Drug Administration. Moderna COVID-19 Vaccines. FDA. Available at: https://www.fda.gov/emergency-preparedness-and-response/coronavirus-disease-2019-covid-19/moderna-covid-19-vaccines. Published 2022. Accessed November 26, 2022.
16. Marrack P, McKee AS, Munks MW. Towards an understanding of the adjuvant action of aluminium. Nat Rev Immunol 2009;9(4):287–93.

17. Ott G, Barchfeld GL, Chernoff D, et al. MF59. Design and evaluation of a safe and potent adjuvant for human vaccines. Pharm Biotechnol 1995;6:277–96.

18. Centers for Disease Control and Prevention. Vaccinate with confidence. CDC. Available at: https://www.cdc.gov/vaccines/partners/vaccinate-with-confidence.html. Published 2019. Accessed December 3, 2022.

19. Control ECfDPa. Vaccine hesitancy. ECDC. Available at: https://www.ecdc.europa.eu/en/immunisation-vaccines/vaccine-hesitancy. Published 2022. Accessed December 3, 2022.

20. World Health Organization. Ten threats to global health in 2019. WHO. Available at: https://www.who.int/news-room/spotlight/ten-threats-to-global-health-in-2019. Published 2022. Accessed November 26, 2022.

21. Salmon DA, Dudley MZ, Glanz JM, et al. Vaccine hesitancy: Causes, consequences, and a call to action. Vaccine 2015;33(Suppl 4):D66–71.

22. Hamel L, Lopes L, Sparks G, et al. KFF COVID-19 Vaccine Monitor: Media and Misinformation. Kaiser Family Foundation. Available at: https://www.kff.org/coronavirus-covid-19/poll-finding/kff-covid-19-vaccine-monitor-media-and-misinformation/. Published 2021. Accessed December 3, 2022.

23. Battarbee AN, Stockwell MS, Varner M, et al. Attitudes Toward COVID-19 Illness and COVID-19 Vaccination among Pregnant Women: A Cross-Sectional Multicenter Study during August-December 2020. Am J Perinatol 2022;39(1):75–83.

24. Shook LL, Kishkovich TP, Edlow AG. Countering COVID-19 Vaccine Hesitancy in Pregnancy: the "4 Cs. Am J Perinatol 2022;39(10):1048–54.

25. Meeting the Challenge of Vaccination Hesitancy. The Aspen Institute, Sabin Vaccine Institute. Sabin-Aspen Vaccine Science & Policy Group Web site. Available at: https://www.sabin.org/app/uploads/2022/04/Sabin-Aspen-report-2020_Meeting-the-Challenge-of-Vaccine-Hesitancy.pdf. Published 2020. Accessed Dec 6, 2022.

26. Basch CH, Zybert P, Reeves R, et al. What do popular YouTube(TM) videos say about vaccines? Child Care Health Dev 2017;43(4):499–503.

27. Puri N, Coomes EA, Haghbayan H, et al. Social media and vaccine hesitancy: new updates for the era of COVID-19 and globalized infectious diseases. Hum Vaccin Immunother 2020;16(11):2586–93.

28. Li HO, Bailey A, Huynh D, et al. YouTube as a source of information on COVID-19: a pandemic of misinformation? BMJ Glob Health 2020;5(5):e002604.

29. Yuan X, Schuchard RJ, Crooks AT. Examining Emergent Communities and Social Bots Within the Polarized Online Vaccination Debate in Twitter. Social Media + Society 2019;5(3). 2056305119865465.

30. Blankenship EB, Goff ME, Yin J, et al. Sentiment, Contents, and Retweets: A Study of Two Vaccine-Related Twitter Datasets. Perm J 2018;22:17–138.

31. Gunaratne K, Coomes EA, Haghbayan H. Temporal trends in anti-vaccine discourse on. Twitter. Vaccine 2019;37(35):4867–71.

32. Broniatowski DA, Jamison AM, Qi S, et al. Weaponized Health Communication: Twitter Bots and Russian Trolls Amplify the Vaccine Debate. Am J Public Health 2018;108(10):1378–84.

33. Madara JL. AMA vaccines letter to social media tech companies (ama-assn.org), 2019, American Medical Association. Available at: https://www.ama-assn.org/system/files/2019-03/madara-vaccination-letter.pdf.

34. American College of Obstetricians and Gynecologists' Committee on Adolescent Health Care ACoOaGI. Infectious Disease, and Public Health Preparedness Expert Work Group,. Human Papillomavirus Vaccination: ACOG Committee Opinion, Number 809. Obstet Gynecol 2020;136(2):e15–21.

35. Meites E, Szilagyi PG, Chesson HW, et al. Human Papillomavirus Vaccination for Adults: Updated Recommendations of the Advisory Committee on Immunization Practices. MMWR Morb Mortal Wkly Rep 2019;68(32):698–702.

36. Nicol AF, Andrade CV, Russomano FB, et al. HPV vaccines: a controversial issue? Braz J Med Biol Res 2016;49(5):e5060.

37. Bednarczyk RA. Addressing HPV vaccine myths: practical information for healthcare providers. Hum Vaccin Immunother 2019;15(7–8):1628–38.

38. Szilagyi PG, Albertin CS, Gurfinkel D, et al. Prevalence and characteristics of HPV vaccine hesitancy among parents of adolescents across the US. Vaccine 2020;38(38):6027–37.

39. Williams CL, Walker TY, Elam-Evans LD, et al. Factors associated with not receiving HPV vaccine among adolescents by metropolitan statistical area status, United States, National Immunization Survey-Teen, 2016-2017. Hum Vaccin Immunother 2020;16(3):562–72.

40. Kasting ML, Shapiro GK, Rosberger Z, et al. Tempest in a teapot: A systematic review of HPV vaccination and risk compensation research. Hum Vaccin Immunother 2016;12(6):1435–50.

41. Arnheim-Dahlström L, Pasternak B, Svanström H, et al. Autoimmune, neurological, and venous thromboembolic adverse events after immunisation of adolescent girls with quadrivalent human papillomavirus vaccine in Denmark and Sweden: cohort study. Bmj 2013;347:f5906.

42. DeStefano F, Bodenstab HM, Offit PA. Principal Controversies in Vaccine Safety in the United States. Clin Infect Dis 2019;69(4):726–31.

43. Scheller NM, Svanström H, Pasternak B, et al. Quadrivalent HPV vaccination and risk of multiple sclerosis and other demyelinating diseases of the central nervous system. JAMA 2015;313(1):54–61.

44. McRee AL, Gilkey MB, Dempsey AF. HPV vaccine hesitancy: findings from a statewide survey of health care providers. J Pediatr Health Care 2014;28(6):541–9.

45. Grohskopf LA, Blanton LH, Ferdinands JM, et al. Prevention and Control of Seasonal Influenza with Vaccines: Recommendations of the Advisory Committee on Immunization Practices - United States, 2022-23 Influenza Season. MMWR Recomm Rep (Morb Mortal Wkly Rep) 2022;71(1):1–28.

46. Harper SA, Fukuda K, Uyeki TM, et al. Prevention and control of influenza. Recommendations of the Advisory Committee on Immunization Practices (ACIP). MMWR Recomm Rep (Morb Mortal Wkly Rep) 2005;54(Rr-8):1–40.

47. Centers for Disease Control and Prevention. Healthy People 2020 Data. CDC. Available at: https://www.cdc.gov/nchs/healthy_people/hp2020/hp2020_data. htm. Published 2019. Accessed December 4, 2022.

48. Kerr S, Van Bennekom CM, Mitchell AA. Influenza Vaccination Coverage During Pregnancy - Selected Sites, United States, 2005-06 Through 2013-14 Influenza Vaccine Seasons. MMWR Morb Mortal Wkly Rep 2016;65(48):1370–3.

49. Ramey-Collier KL, Okunbor JI, Lunn SR, et al. Prenatal Vaccination Patterns among Birthing Individuals with History of Preterm Birth in the Pre- and Post-COVID Era. Am J Perinatol 2023. https://doi.org/10.1055/s-0042-1760432.

50. Zerbo O, Ray GT, Zhang L, et al. Individual and Neighborhood Factors Associated With Failure to Vaccinate Against Influenza During Pregnancy. Am J Epidemiol 2020;189(11):1379–88.

51. Sheffield JS, Greer LG, Rogers VL, et al. Effect of influenza vaccination in the first trimester of pregnancy. Obstet Gynecol 2012;120(3):532–7.

52. Nordin JD, Kharbanda EO, Benitez GV, et al. Maternal safety of trivalent inactivated influenza vaccine in pregnant women. Obstet Gynecol 2013;121(3): 519–25.

53. Kharbanda EO, Vazquez-Benitez G, Romitti PA, et al. First Trimester Influenza Vaccination and Risks for Major Structural Birth Defects in Offspring. J Pediatr 2017;187:234–9.e234.

54. McMillan M, Porritt K, Kralik D, et al. Influenza vaccination during pregnancy: a systematic review of fetal death, spontaneous abortion, and congenital malformation safety outcomes. Vaccine 2015;33(18):2108–17.

55. Polyzos KA, Konstantelias AA, Pitsa CE, et al. Maternal Influenza Vaccination and Risk for Congenital Malformations: A Systematic Review and Meta-analysis. Obstet Gynecol 2015;126(5):1075–84.

56. Hviid A, Svanström H, Mølgaard-Nielsen D, et al. Association Between Pandemic Influenza A(H1N1) Vaccination in Pregnancy and Early Childhood Morbidity in Offspring. JAMA Pediatr 2017;171(3):239–48.

57. Bratton KN, Wardle MT, Orenstein WA, et al. Maternal influenza immunization and birth outcomes of stillbirth and spontaneous abortion: a systematic review and meta-analysis. Clin Infect Dis 2015;60(5):e11–9.

58. Legge A, Dodds L, MacDonald NE, et al. Rates and determinants of seasonal influenza vaccination in pregnancy and association with neonatal outcomes. CMAJ (Can Med Assoc J) 2014;186(4):E157–64.

59. Steinhoff MC, Omer SB, Roy E, et al. Neonatal outcomes after influenza immunization during pregnancy: a randomized controlled trial. CMAJ (Can Med Assoc J) 2012;184(6):645–53.

60. Demicheli V, Jefferson T, Al-Ansary LA, et al. Vaccines for preventing influenza in healthy adults. Cochrane Database Syst Rev 2014;3:Cd001269.

61. Demicheli V, Jefferson T, Ferroni E, et al. Vaccines for preventing influenza in healthy adults. Cochrane Database Syst Rev 2018;2(2):Cd001269.

62. Omer SB, Clark DR, Madhi SA, et al. Efficacy, duration of protection, birth outcomes, and infant growth associated with influenza vaccination in pregnancy: a pooled analysis of three randomised controlled trials. Lancet Respir Med 2020;8(6):597–608.

63. Schmid P, Rauber D, Betsch C, et al. Barriers of Influenza Vaccination Intention and Behavior - A Systematic Review of Influenza Vaccine Hesitancy, 2005 - 2016. PLoS One 2017;12(1):e0170550.

64. Shavell VI, Moniz MH, Gonik B, et al. Influenza immunization in pregnancy: overcoming patient and health care provider barriers. Am J Obstet Gynecol 2012; 207(3 Suppl):S67–74.

65. Adeyanju GC, Engel E, Koch L, et al. Determinants of influenza vaccine hesitancy among pregnant women in Europe: a systematic review. Eur J Med Res 2021;26(1):116.

66. Joint statement of the American Academy of Pediatrics (AAP) and the United States Public Health Service (USPHS). Pediatrics 1999;104(3 Pt 1):568–9.

67. Taylor LE, Swerdfeger AL, Eslick GD. Vaccines are not associated with autism: an evidence-based meta-analysis of case-control and cohort studies. Vaccine 2014;32(29):3623–9.

68. Price CS, Thompson WW, Goodson B, et al. Prenatal and infant exposure to thimerosal from vaccines and immunoglobulins and risk of autism. Pediatrics 2010;126(4):656–64.

69. Liang JL, Tiwari T, Moro P, et al. Prevention of Pertussis, Tetanus, and Diphtheria with Vaccines in the United States: Recommendations of the Advisory

Committee on Immunization Practices (ACIP). MMWR Recomm Rep (Morb Mortal Wkly Rep) 2018;67(2):1–44.

70. World Health Organization: Initiatiaves. "Maternal and Neonatal Tetanus Elimination (MNTE)". Available at: https://www.who.int/initiatives/maternal-and-neonatal-tetanus-elimination-(mnte).

71. Centers for Disease Control and Prevention. Diphtheria, Tetanus, and Pertussis Vaccine Recommendations. CDC. Available at: https://www.cdc.gov/vaccines/hcp/vis/vis-statements/dtap.pdf. Published 2022. Accessed December 4, 2022.

72. Committee Opinion No. 718: Update on Immunization and Pregnancy: Tetanus, Diphtheria, and Pertussis Vaccination. Obstet Gynecol 2017;130(3):e153–7.

73. Tseng HF, Sy LS, Ackerson BK, et al. Safety of tetanus, diphtheria, acellular pertussis (Tdap) vaccination during pregnancy. Vaccine 2022;40(32):4503–12.

74. Munoz FM, Bond NH, Maccato M, et al. Safety and immunogenicity of tetanus diphtheria and acellular pertussis (Tdap) immunization during pregnancy in mothers and infants: a randomized clinical trial. JAMA 2014;311(17):1760–9.

75. Kahn KE, Razzaghi H, Jatlaoui TC, et al. Flu and Tdap Vaccination Coverage Among Pregnant Women – United States, April 2021. CDC. Available at: https://www.cdc.gov/flu/fluvaxview/pregnant-women-apr2021.htm. Published 2021. Accessed December 5, 2022..

76. Chamberlain AT, Seib K, Ault KA, et al. Factors Associated with Intention to Receive Influenza and Tetanus, Diphtheria, and Acellular Pertussis (Tdap) Vaccines during Pregnancy: A Focus on Vaccine Hesitancy and Perceptions of Disease Severity and Vaccine Safety. PLoS Curr 2015;7.

77. Cheng PJ, Huang SY, Shaw SW, et al. Factors influencing women's decisions regarding pertussis vaccine: A decision-making study in the Postpartum Pertussis Immunization Program of a teaching hospital in Taiwan. Vaccine 2010;28(34):5641–7.

78. Gynecologists ACoOa. ACOG and SMFM recommend COVID-19 vaccination for pregnant individuals. ACOG. https://www.acog.org/news/news-releases/2021/07/acog-smfm-recommend-covid-19-vaccination-for-pregnant-individuals. Published 2021. Accessed December 7, 2022.

79. Centers for Disease Control and Prevention. COVID-19 Vaccination for Pregnant People to Prevent Serious Illness, Deaths, and Adverse Pregnancy Outcomes from COVID-19. CDC. Available at: https://emergency.cdc.gov/han/2021/han00453.asp. Published 2021. Accessed December 7, 2022.

80. Centers for Disease Control and Prevention. COVID-19 Vaccines While Pregnant or Breastfeeding. CDC. Available at: https://www.cdc.gov/coronavirus/2019-ncov/vaccines/recommendations/pregnancy.html#:~:text=COVID%2D19%20vaccines%20do%20not,are%20pregnant%20or%20their%20babies. Published 2022. Accessed December 7, 2022.

81. Centers for Disease Control and Prevention. COVID-19 Vaccinations in the United States. CDC. Available at: https://covid.cdc.gov/covid-data-tracker/#vaccinations_vacc-total-admin-rate-total. Published 2022. Accessed September 3, 2022.

82. Irwin A. What it will take to vaccinate the world against COVID-19. Nature 2021;592(7853):176–8.

83. Holder J. Vaccinations around the world. 12, 2022, 2022. The New York Times December 12, 2022. Available at: https://www.nytimes.com/interactive/2021/world/covid-vaccinations-tracker.html.

84. Kachikis A, Englund JA, Covelli I, et al. Analysis of Vaccine Reactions After COVID-19 Vaccine Booster Doses Among Pregnant and Lactating Individuals. JAMA Netw Open 2022;5(9):e2230495.

85. Shook LL, Edlow AG. Safety and Efficacy of Coronavirus Disease 2019 (COVID-19) mRNA Vaccines During Lactation. Obstet Gynecol 2023;141(3):483–91.

86. Smith ER, Oakley E, Grandner GW, et al. Adverse maternal, fetal, and newborn outcomes among pregnant women with SARS-CoV-2 infection: an individual participant data meta-analysis. BMJ Glob Health 2023;8(1):e009495.

87. Shimabukuro T. COVID-19 vaccine safety update. CDC. Available at: https://www.cdc.gov/vaccines/acip/meetings/downloads/slides-2021-02/28 03-01/05-covid-Shimabukuro.pdf. Published 2021. Accessed December 7, 2022.

88. Magnus MC, Gjessing HK, Eide HN, et al. Covid-19 Vaccination during Pregnancy and First-Trimester Miscarriage. N Engl J Med 2021;385(21):2008–10.

89. Collier AY, McMahan K, Yu J, et al. Immunogenicity of COVID-19 mRNA Vaccines in Pregnant and Lactating Women. JAMA 2021;325(23):2370–80.

90. Fu W, Sivajohan B, McClymont E, et al. Systematic review of the safety, immunogenicity, and effectiveness of COVID-19 vaccines in pregnant and lactating individuals and their infants. Int J Gynaecol Obstet 2022;156(3):406–17.

91. Schaler L, Wingfield M. COVID-19 vaccine - can it affect fertility? Ir J Med Sci 2022;191(5):2185–7.

92. Zaçe D, La Gatta E, Petrella L, et al. The impact of COVID-19 vaccines on fertility-A systematic review and meta-analysis. Vaccine 2022;40(42):6023–34.

93. Oliver S. Risk/Benefit assessment of thrombotic thrombocytopenic events after Janssen COVID-19 vaccines: Applying Evidence to Recommendation Framework. CDC. 2021. Available at: https://www.cdc.gov/vaccines/acip/meetings/downloads/slides-2021-04-23/06-COVID-Oliver-508.pdf. Accessed December 1, 2022.

94. Lipkind HS, Vazquez-Benitez G, DeSilva M, et al. Receipt of COVID-19 Vaccine During Pregnancy and Preterm or Small-for-Gestational-Age at Birth - Eight Integrated Health Care Organizations, United States, December 15, 2020-July 22, 2021. MMWR Morb Mortal Wkly Rep 2022;71(1):26–30.

95. Halasa NB, Olson SM, Staat MA. et al. Effectiveness of Maternal Vaccination with mRNA COVID-19 Vaccine During Pregnancy Against COVID-19-Associated Hospitalization in Infants Aged <6 Months - 17 States, July 2021-January 2022. MMWR Morb Mortal Wkly Rep. 2022;71(7):264-270.

96. Shimabukuro T, ACIP COVID-19 Vaccine Safety Update-March 1, 2021. (cdc.gov). Available at: https://www.cdc.gov/vaccines/acip/meetings/downloads/slides-2021-02/28-03-01/05-covid-Shimabukuro.pdf?ftag=YHF4eb9d17.

97. Organization WHO, Coronavirus disease (COVID-19): Pregnancy, childbirth and the postnatal period. 2022. Available at: https://www.who.int/news-room/questions-and-answers/item/coronavirus-disease-covid-19-pregnancy-and-childbirth. Accessed January 3, 2023.

98. Ashby B, Best A. Herd immunity. Curr Biol 2021;31(4):R174–7.

99. Mallory ML, Lindesmith LC, Baric RS. Vaccination-induced herd immunity: Successes and challenges. J Allergy Clin Immunol 2018;142(1):64–6.

100. Esposito S, Stefanelli P, Fry NK, et al. Pertussis Prevention: Reasons for Resurgence, and Differences in the Current Acellular Pertussis Vaccines. Front Immunol 2019;10:1344.

101. Plans-Rubió P. Percentages of Vaccination Coverage Required to Establish Herd Immunity against SARS-CoV-2. Vaccines (Basel) 2022;10:736. https://doi.org/10.3390/vaccines10050736.

102. Beleche T, Ruhter J, Kolbe A, et al. COVID-19 vaccine hesitancy: demographic factors, geographic patterns, and changes over time. 2021;27.
103. de Beaumont Foundation. New poll reveals most effective language to improve COVID-19 vaccine acceptance. de Beaumont Foundation. Available at: https://debeaumont.org/changing-the-covid-conversation/vaccineacceptance/. Published 2020. Accessed November 12, 2022.
104. Marzo RR, Su TT, Ismail R, et al. Digital health literacy for COVID-19 vaccination and intention to be immunized: A cross sectional multi-country study among the general adult population. Front Public Health 2022;10:998234.
105. Soh QR, Oh LYJ, Chow EPF, et al. HIV Testing Uptake According to Opt-In, Opt-Out or Risk-Based Testing Approaches: a Systematic Review and Meta-Analysis. Curr HIV AIDS Rep 2022;19(5):375–83.
106. Blalock SJ, Reyna VF. Using fuzzy-trace theory to understand and improve health judgments, decisions, and behaviors: A literature review. Health Psychol 2016;35(8):781–92.
107. Pinterest Newsroom. Bringing authoritative vaccine results to Pinterest search. 2019. Available at: https://newsroom.pinterest.com/en/post/bringing-authoritative-vaccine-results-to-pinterest-search. Accessed December 9, 2022.
108. McMillan R, Hernandez D. Pinterest Blocks Vaccination Searches in Move to Control the Conversation. Wall Street Journal 2019;20:2019.
109. Monika Bickert V. Global Policy Management. Meta Newsroom, "Combatting Vaccine Misinformation. Available at: https://www.hhs.gov/vaccines/vaccines-national-strategic-plan/index.html. Published 2020. Accessed December 20, 2022.
110. Harvey D. Helping you find reliable public health information on Twitter. Twitter. Available at: https://blog.twitter.com/en_us/topics/company/2019/helping-you-find-reliable-public-health-information-on-twitter. Published 2019. Accessed May 20, 2019.
111. At home #WithMe. YouTube Web Site Web site. Available at: https://www.youtube.com/channel/UCK8qVjkRMl1lRcYp6_W_1qw. Accessed December 6, 2022.
112. Committee Opinion No. 664: Refusal of Medically Recommended Treatment During Pregnancy. Obstet Gynecol 2016;127(6):e175–82.
113. Callender D. Vaccine hesitancy: More than a movement. Hum Vaccin Immunother 2016;12(9):2464–8.

Respiratory Syncytial Virus—An Update for Prenatal and Primary Health Providers

Alisa B. Kachikis, MD, MSc[a],*, Hye Cho, BS[b], Janet A. Englund, MD[c]

KEYWORDS

- Respiratory syncytial virus • RSV • Pneumonia
- Lower respiratory tract infection (LRTI) • Upper respiratory infection (URI)

KEY POINTS

- Respiratory syncytial virus (RSV) infection is a significant cause of morbidity and mortality among infants aged younger than 1 year, adults aged 65 years or older, and immunocompromised persons.
- Limited data exist on RSV infection in pregnancy but studies suggest RSV can cause severe illness, particularly in conjunction with comorbidities, chronic lung disease, and co-infection with other viruses or bacteria.
- Treatment options are currently limited but strides are being made in developing vaccines for maternal immunization and monoclonal antibodies for disease prevention.
- Further researches on RSV pathogenesis, infection prevalence, and disease burden in reproductive age and pregnant individuals are needed.

INTRODUCTION

Respiratory syncytial virus (RSV) is, in addition to SARS-CoV-2 and influenza, one of the most important respiratory pathogens affecting women's health. Although RSV typically affects the extremes of age, the RSV surge in 2022 was described as being one of the worst seasonal surges in recent years. RSV overwhelmed children's hospitals and pediatric care units in the United States and brought RSV infection prevention into the news cycle and mainstream medical discourse.[1] Novel vaccines and monoclonal antibodies have been developed against RSV, utilizing new technology and knowledge advances gained before and after coronavirus disease 2019 (COVID-19) vaccine

[a] Department of Obstetrics & Gynecology, University of Washington, 1959 Northeast Pacific Street, Box 356460, Seattle, WA 98195, USA; [b] SUNY Upstate Medical University, Syracuse, NY, USA; [c] Department of Pediatrics, Seattle Children's Hospital Pediatric Infectious Diseases, Seattle Children's Hospital Research Institute, University of Washington, Seattle, WA, USA
* Corresponding author.
E-mail address: abk26@uw.edu

Obstet Gynecol Clin N Am 50 (2023) 421–437
https://doi.org/10.1016/j.ogc.2023.02.011
0889-8545/23/© 2023 Elsevier Inc. All rights reserved.
obgyn.theclinics.com

development. These RSV vaccines have the potential to harness maternal immunization and transplacental antibody transfer for the prevention of RSV infection in neonates and young infants. However, knowledge gaps and areas for research within women's health are becoming more apparent.[2,3] It is more important than ever for women's health providers to have a basic understanding of RSV and infection prevention to optimize clinical discussions and recommendations in the context of pregnancy and preventive care, especially in light of potential new vaccines and therapeutics for pregnancy.

RESPIRATORY SYNCYTIAL VIRUS

Human RSV is an enveloped RNA virus in the Pneumoviridae family, with 2 strains, group A and group B.[4] Human metapneumovirus is the most closely related human virus to RSV. RSV consists of a nucleocapsid within a lipid envelope that contains transmembrane surface glycoprotein spikes[5] (**Fig. 1**). Two transmembrane surface proteins, G (attachment) and F (fusion), are important for viral infectivity and are antigens of interest for antibody-mediated neutralization.[5] The G protein helps the RSV virus attach to respiratory epithelial and immune cells. After attachment, the prefusion F protein undergoes structural changes. The postfusion F protein initiates viral entry by fusing the viral envelope to the host cell membrane. The F protein also fuses host cells to form syncytia.[5,6]

Transmission

Infection with RSV is mediated through droplets and by touching objects that have been contaminated by viral particles. In addition, large particle aerosols generated by sneezing or coughing may transmit RSV within a 3-ft radius.[7] The incubation period is around 2 to 8 days with natural infection. Shedding duration typically ranges from 7 to 10 days but virus can occasionally still be found for up to 30 days.[8,9] Higher viral load is associated with increased disease severity.[10,11]

Pathogenesis

RSV infects respiratory epithelial cells, primarily ciliated columnar cells, but also type I and type II pneumocytes and spreads directly from the nasopharynx along the airways.[12,13] In a primary infection, lower respiratory tract infection (LRTI) often manifests

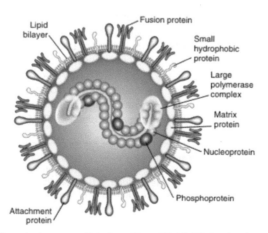

Fig. 1. Structure of respiratory syncytial virus. (*From* Walsh EE, Englund JA. Chapter 158: Respiratory Syncytial Virus. Mandell, Douglas, and Bennett's Principles and Practice of Infectious Diseases. 9th ed: Elsevier; 2020. p. 2093-103.e6; with permission.)

as bronchiolitis in which there is lymphocytic peribronchiolar infiltration and edema followed by proliferation and necrosis of bronchiolar epithelium.[12,14,15] Clinical manifestations of RSV infection, particularly in young infants with small airways, including the characteristic atelectasis resulting from sloughed epithelium, increased mucus secretion, and trapping of air due to partial occlusions of airways. Within a week of RSV illness, some of the bronchiolar epithelium begins to regenerate, although it may take weeks for ciliated cells to recover.[12,14]

Pathogenesis of RSV infection and severity of the disease is thought to be associated with multiple factors including genetics, age of the infant and gestational age at birth, ability of the immune system to fight the infection, whether via maternally derived antibody, monoclonal antibodies or the individual's own immune response. Other factors that are also important include environmental exposures, coinfection with other viruses or bacteria, the person's age, and virulence of the virus itself.[16–18] RSV infection has been associated with increased pathogenicity of *Streptococcus pneumoniae*, and an increase in pneumococcal pneumonia in children is often seen during RSV epidemics.[19] With increased respiratory infection surveillance, codetection of RSV-subtypes and codetection of RSV with various other pathogens have been found to be associated with higher clinical severity.[20–22]

Detection
Laboratory diagnosis is currently best made by reverse-transcriptase polymerase chain reaction (RT-PCR) testing but some rapid diagnostic commercial antigen tests or immunofluorescent antigen detection tests may also be available.[5] The sensitivity of the diagnostic tests depends on the specimen type and viral load. In the outpatient setting, combined throat and nose swabs may improve the RSV detection; however, nasal swabs alone have shown similar detection rates when utilizing sensitive RT-PCR techniques.[23–25]

Respiratory Syncytial Virus and the Immune System

Maternally derived immunity
Maternally derived RSV-specific IgG is the first line of defense against RSV infection in neonates and infants. Active transplacental transfer of these antibodies occurs during pregnancy through neonatal Fc receptors of syncytiotrophoblast cells in the chorionic villi of the placenta.[26,27] Maternally derived RSV-specific antibodies have a relatively short half-life of 28 to 40 days but have been demonstrated to be efficiently transferred across the placenta to the fetus in multiple studies from around the globe.[28,29] Most of these studies have found associations between maternal antibody concentrations and neutralizing function and protection of the infant from severe RSV illness.[29–32] An early US study from 1981 demonstrated that higher levels of neutralizing antibody in cord blood was correlated with older age of the infant at hospitalization for RSV illness.[31] Similarly, a study from Denmark from 2009 found that increases in cord blood neutralizing activity of antibodies was associated with reductions in hospitalization during the first 6 months of life.[32] A more recent study from 2017 showed that antibody concentrations to prefusion-F and G proteins and neutralizing activity were associated with decreased disease severity in the first months of life.[30] In addition to studies on maternal immunization with RSV F-protein vaccines, other prospective studies on monoclonal antibodies in at-risk infants also demonstrate that passively obtained antibody is protective against severe RSV illness.[33,34]

Innate and adaptive immunity
RSV infection triggers a rapid and vigorous innate immune response in the respiratory epithelium.[5,35,36] Interactions between RSV and Toll-like receptors triggers

inflammatory cytokines and chemokines resulting in recruitment of macrophages, mononuclear cells, natural killer cells and eosinophils.[37] In addition, dendritic cells are recruited into the nasal mucosa during infection. Concentrations of the innate immune cells and levels of chemokines and cytokines have been found to correlate with disease pathogenesis and severity.[36]

The adaptive immune response to RSV infection depends on host and viral factors. In a primary infection, immunoglobulin (Ig) M antibody is produced within days but its presence is transient. IgG can be detected in the second week after infection and peaks in week 4. Following approximately 3 infections and reinfections in young children, IgG titers are similar to those found in adults.[18] IgG antibodies are developed to many of the RSV proteins, including surface glycoproteins F and G.[38] In adults, natural infection results in a 4-fold increase in antibodies that returns to previous levels after about 2 years following the infection.[39] In general, higher concentrations of antibody have been found to correlate to higher resistance to infection but there is no defined threshold of protection against risk for infection, severity of illness or recovery in both children and adults.[40,41]

Other antibodies including RSV-specific IgA and IgE can be produced in response to RSV infection. IgA can be found in nasal secretions in primary and secondary infections, and although associated with viral clearance, IgA-specific memory B cell induction seems to be impaired, resulting in increased reinfection.[41–43] IgE may also be produced transiently in some cases and higher levels of IgE has been associated with increased disease severity and wheezing with later episodes of wheezing.[44]

Cell-mediated immunity is also important for viral clearance and disease recovery, and people with cell-mediated immunodeficiencies have more severe disease and viral shedding.[45,46] Multiple inhibitory effects on cell-mediated immunity are at play in RSV disease including inhibition of antiviral interferon gamma signals and helper T-cell responses.[36,47] RSV infection triggers both Th1 and Th2 immune pathways, and the balance between these immune responses is of increasing interest in elucidating RSV pathogenesis. In contrast to Th1 responses, associated with viral clearance and decreased pathology, Th2 responses correlate with increased symptoms including wheezing, disease severity, and inflammation.[48] Young infants, for example, are more likely to be found to have higher Th2-type cytokines in nasal secretions than older infants or children.[49,50]

Clinical Impact—Epidemiology and Disease Burden

Seasonality

Seasonal RSV outbreaks vary somewhat depending on geography and year but are overall consistent over time.[51,52] Globally, RSV epidemics start in the south hemisphere fall and winter, and move to the north hemisphere.[53] The RSV wave typically starts in the Southern Hemisphere between the months of March and June and then appears in the Northern Hemispheres around September through December.[51,53,54] RSV seasons usually last 4 to 6 months although shorter or longer seasons can be observed in certain regions and in countries with rainy or humid seasons (**Fig. 2**).[53] RSV seasons can also vary greater depending on global events such as the COVID-19 pandemic when the RSV season was exceptionally light due to other infection prevention measures.[55]

Global impact

From a global perspective, pneumonia and prematurity are the major causes of morbidity and mortality of neonates and children aged younger than 5 years

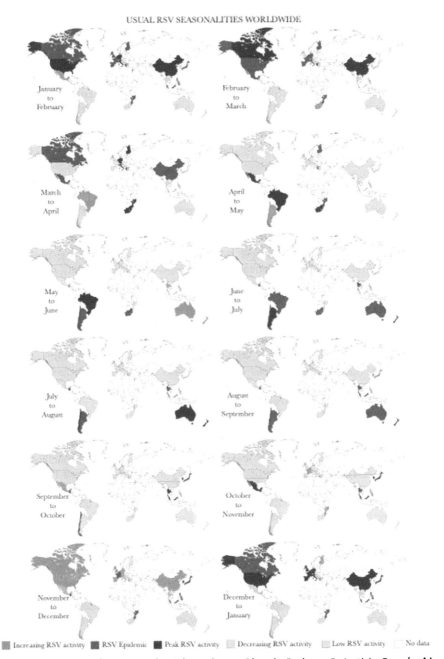

Fig. 2. Country-specific RSV epidemiology. (*From* Obando-Pacheco P, Justicia-Grande AJ, Rivero-Calle I, et al. Respiratory Syncytial Virus Seasonality: A Global Overview. J Infect Dis. 2018;217(9):1356-1364; with permission.)

worldwide, and this is particularly true in Sub-Saharan Africa and Asia.[56] In children aged younger than 5 years, RSV accounts for the majority of LRTI.[57] Therefore, there have been significant global efforts to develop options for RSV prophylaxis in infants worldwide including maternal immunizations to be administered during pregnancy or monoclonal antibodies to be administered to infants after birth.[2,58,59]

Similarly, in older adults aged 65 years or older, RSV accounts for a significant disease burden, particularly in those with comorbidities. However, estimates in adults are limited by the lack of available data from low-income and middle-income countries.[60] A recent meta-analysis of RSV in older adults in high-income countries found that actual disease burden was higher than earlier estimates and generally similar to disease burden due to influenza. This emphasizes the need for improved RSV surveillance systems particularly in low-income and middle-income countries and RSV prevention and prophylaxis in the population group of adults aged 65 years or older.[61]

Infants and children

RSV is the leading causative pathogen among infants and young children with LRTI. It is expected that 70% of children aged younger than 12 months will be infected with RSV and nearly all children will be infected with RSV by 24 months.[62–64] In 2019, it was estimated that 3.6 million hospital admissions were due to RSV-associated LRTI among children aged younger than 5 years and, among these, there were 26,300 RSV-related LRTI in-hospital deaths.[57] However, the mortality rate is even higher when considering community-based mortality due to RVS illness. The RSV-attributable overall deaths were estimated to be 101,400 among children aged younger than 5 years in 2019.[57] This number make RSV a major cause of mortality in this age group and a significant burden on the health-care system.

After the COVID-19 pandemic started in the United States in 2020, RSV infection rates declined to very low levels. Although infection prevention methods such as face masks, hand-washing, social distancing, and stay-at-home orders helped to contain the spread of many infections, they did not allow for children to be exposed to RSV and develop protective immunity.[65] Since the relaxation of COVID-19 restrictions, there has been an unprecedented increase in pediatric RSV hospitalizations— far more than the usual number of children who previously required hospitalization due to RSV LRTI during the RSV season before the COVID19 pandemic.[66]

In children aged younger than 1 year, RSV is the main cause of bronchiolitis and pneumonia.[67] Two to 4 days of upper respiratory tract symptoms are typically followed by lower respiratory tract symptoms in infants with RSV bronchiolitis. Upper respiratory tract symptoms include fever, runny nose, and nasal congestion. Lower respiratory tract symptoms can present as increasing cough, rapid and labored breathing, dyspnea, and difficulty feeding. In addition, otitis media can commonly present in children with RSV infections.[68] In 74% of children with acute otitis media, RSV was detected in the middle ear fluid.[68]

Infants with RSV-related LRTI may continue to develop wheezing throughout their early childhood years, which may even persist into adulthood,[69] although the causality of RSV influencing the development of asthma remains under debate. Studies have further suggested an association between RSV infection in infancy and future development of asthma, allergies, and poor pulmonary function, with significant impact on quality of life in the future.[70]

Pregnant individuals

There are limited data on the prevalence and significance of RSV infections and disease in pregnant people. A prospective community-based study from Nepal found the incidence of RSV illness among their pregnant participants to be 0.4% (14 of 3693 women) from 2011 to 2014. Of these, 7 (50%) sought medical care for their RSV illness.[71] Additionally, among 7 cases of postpartum RSV infection in this study,

4 (57%) also involved the RSV infection of the infant.[71] A case series from the United States in 2014 involving 3 pregnant individuals with RSV infection reported that 2 were hospitalized and required intubation while the third had a self-limited infection with out-patient management.[72] These cases highlight that RSV infection during pregnancy may lead to severe maternal disease. In addition, in this case series, all 3 pregnant individuals had either preexisting lung conditions (ie, asthma) or coinfections with influenza A (H1N1) or group A streptococcus.[72] Finally, a prospective cohort study from 2015 to 2016 in the United States demonstrated that 10% of pregnant participants with acute respiratory illness had PCR-confirmed RSV infection.[73] Among these participants, the most common symptoms reported were cough, congestion, and sore throat. Four individuals had symptoms consistent with LRTI (ie, shortness of breath or wheezing). In this study, most individuals with PCR-confirmed RSV infection were seen in the prenatal care clinic during their illness. One participant with twin pregnancy in the third trimester required hospitalization and a course of oral antibiotics for LRTI.[73]

Given the importance of RSV as a pathogen among high-risk adults, RSV infection should be considered in cases of severe ARI or LRTI among pregnant individuals and especially among those with other morbidities such as preexisting pulmonary conditions.[74] RSV coinfection should be considered in cases of severe influenza or other respiratory infections.[72,74] Based on data demonstrating adverse outcomes with other respiratory infections during pregnancy such as influenza or SARS-CoV-2,[75,76] pregnant individuals with RSV infection should be monitored for the development of severe maternal disease with the need for additional supportive care.

Adults aged 65 years and above

Adults aged older than 65 years and those with chronic diseases or immunosuppression are at high risk for severe RSV infection. Although RSV is a leading cause of viral illness and death in children aged younger than 1 year, RSV-associated mortality rates are greater in the elderly population. One study found that more than 78% of the respiratory and circulatory deaths related to RSV were among those aged 65 years or older.[77] In the United States, approximately 60,000 to 120,000 older adults are hospitalized due to RSV every year and among those aged 65 years and older, there are 11,000 annual RSV-related deaths.[74]

Clinically, RSV presents very similarly to other respiratory viruses in the elderly population and generally begins with common cold-like symptoms, including cough, sore throat, rhinitis, and dyspnea.[78] Outcomes may vary from asymptomatic infection to respiratory failure and even death.[78] Because of its similar presentation to other respiratory viruses, multiple molecular, serologic, and culture methods may be needed to make a conclusive diagnosis.[74] Some factors that may explain the increased RSV severity among older adults include age-related decline in immune and pulmonary function. Preexisting comorbidities may also explain RSV severity in this population. However, further research into RSV susceptibility in this population is needed because the elderly have not been found to have a marked defect in humoral immunity, and there are likely other significant contributing factors.[79]

The risk of developing severe RSV illness is high among immunocompromised patients as well, such as patients receiving solid-organ transplant (SOT) and hematopoietic cell transplantation (HCT). One study reported RSV as being responsible for 7% to 33% of LRTI-associated deaths in HCT recipients.[79,80] One long-term complication affecting almost 10% of immunocompromised patients with RSV is bronchiolitis obliterans syndrome.[81] In lung transplant patients, the rate is even higher at 50%.[81] Although older adults and immunocompromised patients remain a highly vulnerable group at risk for severe RSV illness, new treatments and supportive care may be helpful in improving RSV mortality rates.

Treatment and Prevention

Antiviral medications

Ribavirin, a nucleoside analog, is currently the only United States Food and Drug Administration (FDA)-approved antiviral therapy for use against RSV. Although it is only licensed for infants and young children, ribavirin is also being prescribed for the treatment of severely immunocompromised adults. Delivered in an aerosolized form, ribavirin exhibits in vitro activity against RSV by inhibiting messenger RNA expression and viral protein synthesis.[82]

Although ribavirin remains an option for treatment, there is inadequate evidence regarding its efficacy and safety with conflicting evidence regarding reduction of bronchiolitis incidence in previously healthy children.[83] It is also controversial whether ribavirin treatment decreases the length of hospital stay and need for mechanical ventilation and supplemental oxygen.[83] In addition, potential teratogenicity in pregnant persons and potential airway disease is a significant concern with the use of ribavirin, not only for the patient but also for health-care providers with inhalation exposure to ribavirin.[84] High costs of ribavirin also contribute to its slow adoption as an RSV treatment option, and its use is therefore restricted to severe cases.[85]

Due to the route of administration and high costs of aerosol ribavirin, there has been an increased interest in the oral form due to its lower costs and easier administration. Because oral ribavirin has been used in patients with hepatitis C virus infections, there is more data to support its tolerability.[5] With regards to mortality and progression to LRTI, in observational trials, there was no substantial considerable difference between the 2 routes of administration. Although oral ribavirin seems to be an effective substitute for the aerosolized version, further studies are needed to conclusively support the switch.

Ribavirin is not recommended in pregnancy or for male partners of pregnant individuals because animal studies have shown significant teratogenicity. The Ribavirin Pregnancy Registry (NCT00114712) was established in 2003 to evaluate pregnancy outcomes after Ribavirin exposure.[86] Results of this study published in 2022 show that although the 95% confidence interval around congenital anomaly rate of pregnancies exposed to ribavirin exceeds the Metropolitan Atlanta Congenital Defects Program (MACDP), no patterns indicative of teratogenic mechanism were found. Given small sample size, results must be interpreted with caution.[86]

Monoclonal Antibodies

Monoclonal antibody therapy directed against the RSV F-protein has been shown to provide effective protection against severe RSV illness. Palivizumab is an RSV-specific IgG1 monoclonal antibody that is prophylactically administered to preterm and high-risk infants. Palivizumab works by targeting site II of the F (fusion) protein of RSV.[87] The American Academy of Pediatrics only recommends palivizumab for those who have an increased risk of severe RSV disease and are aged younger than 1 year, including those born prematurely before 29 weeks' gestation, and infants with congenital heart disease or chronic lung disease.[88] The IMpact-RSV clinical trial demonstrated that high-risk infants who were given palivizumab prophylaxis had a 4.8% RSV hospitalization rate, which was 5.8% lower than infants in the placebo recipient group.[89]

Motavizumab, a second-generation monoclonal antibody derived from palivizumab that also targets the F protein of RSV demonstrated greater RSV neutralization activity than palivizumab.[87] However, it failed to show improved outcomes compared with palivizumab while associated with a greater number of cases of cutaneous hypersensitivity reactions. Therefore, the FDA rejected motavizumab in 2010.[87]

A newer monoclonal antibody, nirsevimab, was recently accepted for review by the FDA. Nirsevimab is the first single-dose prophylaxis not only for preterm and high-risk infants but also for all infants regardless of health status and gestational age at birth and is targeted against site 0 of the RSV F protein. Nirsevimab has an extended half-life of up to 6 months.[90] Clinical trials with nirsevimab have shown promising safety and efficacy data; there were no serious hypersensitivity reactions accompanying administration, and side effects potentially associated with nirsevimab only occurred in 1% of infants. Results from the *MELODY* trial demonstrated that a single dose of nirsevimab was effective in reducing RSV-related LRTI in infants by 74.5%.[91]

Vaccines

There are currently no available vaccines against RSV for use in any population group, although multiple vaccines against RSV are currently in development and clinical trials (**Fig. 3**).[92] New vaccine candidates include subunit, particle, vector-based, and live-attenuated platforms.[5] In addition, recent advances in technology have led to a better understanding of the RSV F-protein and design of vaccines with a stable prefusion form of the F-protein.[5]

Given high disease burden, the main population groups targeted for vaccine development are young infants who are particularly at risk for severe RSV disease in the first months of life. Protecting young infants could include administration of a vaccine in the early weeks of life or maternal immunization during pregnancy, similar to the approach

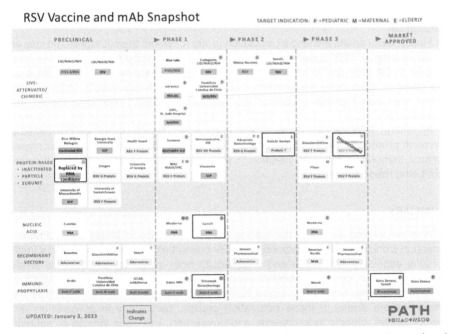

Fig. 3. Snapshot of RSV vaccine and monoclonal antibody trials in process. (*Reproduced from* the PATH website. RSV Vaccine and mAb Snapshot. Published January 2023. Available at https://www.path.org/resources/rsv-vaccine-and-mab-snapshot/.)

taken with influenza and acellular pertussis during pregnancy.[93–95] As seen with other vaccines administered during pregnancy, boosting maternal RSV antibodies using an RSV F protein-based vaccine may result in higher neonatal antibody concentrations and help protect infants until they are older and at lower risk for severe RSV illness. Two large clinical trials for maternal immunization with RSV vaccines have been conducted. Results of a large international trial where 4636 pregnant women were randomized to receive a nanoparticle F protein vaccine candidate versus placebo (Novavax, Gaithersburg, MD) showed up to 90 days of life 39.4% vaccine efficacy in decreasing RSV-associated medically significant LRTI in infants up to 90 days of life compared with placebo, 48.3% vaccine efficacy in preventing RSV-associated LRTI with severe hypoxemia compared with placebo, and 44.4% vaccine efficacy in preventing hospitalization for RSV-associated LRTI.[96] Although the results for this RSV F protein nanoparticle vaccine did not meet prespecified success criterion for vaccine efficacy, the results suggest benefit for infants via RSV vaccine in pregnancy.[96] Another large phase 3 clinical trial recently concluded their enrollment in the United States in 2022 and announced that their maternal vaccine was 82% effective in preventing severe RSV-associated LRTI in infants in the first 90 days of life and was 69% effective in the first 6 months of life (NCT04424316).[97] These results, however, have not yet been published. Nevertheless, multiple pharmaceutical companies are working on developing additional vaccines or monoclonal antibodies against RSV, and it is expected that regulatory decisions will be made in United States in the near future.[98]

Another strategy for older infants or children is vaccination with live-attenuated vaccines against RSV.[99,100] Vaccine candidates for this population group are administered intranasally and contain gene modifications improve attenuation and immunogenic responses.[100] One advantage of this approach is induction of nasal IgA production and cellular immune responses in addition to serum antibody production.[5]

Finally, older adults are also a population group for whom there is significant interest in developing an RSV subunit F or G vaccine. Although subunit vaccines have been shown to be safe and immunogenic in past studies, vaccine trials in adults aged 65 years or older have demonstrated disappointing efficacy results until recently, when prefusion F protein vaccines are reportedly showing promising results (not published).[5]

In general, RSV vaccine development is impeded by lack of defined correlated of immune protection, difficulty determining clinical endpoints for trials and decreased natural immunity after RSV infection.[59] However, with new technology, advances are being made in this field.

SUMMARY

RSV is recognized as one of the leading causes of childhood illness and pulmonary infection worldwide. New approaches to RSV prevention have important clinical implications especially for infants and older adults both on global and national levels. Although data on the impact of RSV infection in reproductive-age and pregnant individuals is lacking, small prospective studies and case series indicate that RSV can cause severe illness in these population groups, particularly in conjunction with comorbidities, chronic lung disease, and coinfection with other viruses or bacteria. In terms of prevention options, monoclonal antibodies such as palivizumab and nirsevimab have shown promising results in preventing severe LRTI in infants. Although there are no vaccines currently approved for any population groups, ongoing clinical trials of the RSV vaccines in development, particularly those on maternal immunization with RSV vaccine during pregnancy, have shown favorable outcomes.

Despite advances in this field, further research regarding RSV disease pathogenesis, the immune response, prevention, and treatment is needed. Specifically, there is insufficient knowledge about the prevalence of RSV infection in pregnancy and the effects of RSV in reproductive-age and pregnant individuals. Further research in this population is particularly of interest given the promising results of maternal RSV vaccines in pregnancy and antibody titers in infants.

Although RSV has previously not been well known in obstetrics and gynecology, advances in vaccine development and interest in maternal immunization are propelling RSV vaccine in pregnancy to the forefront of national health discourse. In addition, there is significant interest in developing an RSV vaccine for routine preventive care adults aged 65 years or older. It will become more and more important for prenatal and primary care providers to be familiar with RSV and prevention options in order to provide counseling in the near future.

CLINICS CARE POINTS

- RSV infection is a significant cause of morbidity and mortality among infants aged younger than 1 year, adults aged 65 years or older and immunocompromised persons.

- Limited data exist on RSV infection in pregnancy but studies suggest RSV can cause severe illness, particularly in conjunction with comorbidities, chronic lung disease, and coinfection with other viruses or bacteria.

- RSV infection should be suspected with symptoms of URI or LRTI in any individual who is pregnant, aged 65 years of age or older, or immunocompromised especially during the late fall and early winter months.

- Laboratory diagnosis is currently best made by RT-PCR of combined nasal-pharyngeal swabs or nasal swabs alone.

- There are no treatment options available for pregnant individuals given concern for potential teratogenicity with ribavirin. Care is largely supportive.

- Strides are being made to develop RSV vaccines, including vaccines for maternal immunization, as well as monoclonal antibodies for disease prevention.

DISCLOSURES

A. Kachikis is an unpaid consultant for GlaxoSmith-Kline and Pfizer. She receives grant support from Pfizer and Merck. J A. Englund is a consultant for Sanofi Pasteur, AstraZeneca, Meissa Vaccines, Pfizer, and Moderna. Research support to Dr Englund's institution is received from Pfizer, GlaxoSmithKline, AstraZeneca, and Merck.

REFERENCES

1. Englund JA. RSV is surging. Progress in preventing it looks promising. Scientic American; 2022 [Available at: https://www.scientificamerican.com/article/rsv-is-surging-progress-in-preventing-it-looks-promising/.
2. Marchant A, Sadarangani M, Garand M, et al. Maternal immunisation: collaborating with mother nature. Lancet Infect Dis 2017;17(7):e197–208.
3. Advancing RSV Maternal Immunization: A Gap Analysis Report, 2018, Seattle https://media.path.org/documents/Advancing_RSV_Maternal_Immunization__A_

Gap_Analysis_Report.pdf?_gl=1*1hh91r2*_ga*NDIxMzg2MDYuMTY3OTMzN
TUxNQ..*_ga_YBSE7ZKDQM*MTY3OTMzNTUxNS4xLjAuMTY3OTMzNTUxNS
4wLjAuMA.

4. Maes P, Amarasinghe GK, Ayllón MA, et al. Taxonomy of the order Mononega-
virales: second update 2018. Arch Virol 2019;164(4):1233–44.

5. Walsh EE, Englund JA. 9th edition. Respiratory syncytial virus. Mandell, Douglas, and Bennett's Principles and Practice of infectious diseases, 158. Elsevier;
2020. p. 2093–103.e6.

6. Goering RV, Dockrell HM, Zimmerman M, et al. Chapter 20: Lower respiratory
tract infections. Mims, . medical microbiology and immunology. 6th edition?0.
Elsevier; 2019. p. 204–33.

7. Hall CB, Douglas RG Jr. Modes of transmission of respiratory syncytial virus.
J Pediatr 1981;99(1):100–3.

8. Johnson KM, Chanock RM, Rifkind D, et al. Respiratory syncytial virus. IV. Correlation of virus shedding, serologic response, and illness in adult volunteers.
JAMA 1961;176:663–7.

9. DeVincenzo JP, Wilkinson T, Vaishnaw A, et al. Viral load drives disease in humans experimentally infected with respiratory syncytial virus. Am J Respir Crit
Care Med 2010;182(10):1305–14.

10. Hall CB, Douglas RG Jr, Geiman JM. Quantitative shedding patterns of respiratory syncytial virus in infants. J Infect Dis 1975;132(2):151–6.

11. Houben ML, Coenjaerts FE, Rossen JW, et al. Disease severity and viral load are
correlated in infants with primary respiratory syncytial virus infection in the community. J Med Virol 2010;82(7):1266–71.

12. Johnson JE, Gonzales RA, Olson SJ, et al. The histopathology of fatal untreated
human respiratory syncytial virus infection. Mod Pathol 2007;20(1):108–19.

13. Welliver TP, Reed JL, Welliver RC, et al. Respiratory syncytial virus and influenza
virus infections: observations from tissues of fatal infant cases. Pediatr Infect Dis
J 2008;27(10 Suppl):S92–6.

14. Welliver TP, Garofalo RP, Hosakote Y, et al. Severe human lower respiratory tract
illness caused by respiratory syncytial virus and influenza virus is characterized
by the absence of pulmonary cytotoxic lymphocyte responses. J Infect Dis
2007;195(8):1126–36.

15. de Souza Costa VH Jr, Baurakiades E, Viola Azevedo ML, et al. Immunohisto-
chemistry analysis of pulmonary infiltrates in necropsy samples of children
with non-pandemic lethal respiratory infections (RSV; ADV; PIV1; PIV2; PIV3;
FLU A; FLU B). J Clin Virol 2014;61(2):211–5.

16. Openshaw PJ, Tregoning JS. Immune responses and disease enhancement
during respiratory syncytial virus infection. Clin Microbiol Rev 2005;18(3):
541–55.

17. Miyairi I, DeVincenzo JP. Human genetic factors and respiratory syncytial virus
disease severity. Clin Microbiol Rev 2008;21(4):686–703.

18. Collins PL, Graham BS. Viral and host factors in human respiratory syncytial virus pathogenesis. J Virol 2008;82(5):2040–55.

19. Weinberger DM, Klugman KP, Steiner CA, et al. Association between respiratory
syncytial virus activity and pneumococcal disease in infants: a time series analysis of US hospitalization data. PLoS Med 2015;12(1):e1001776.

20. Choe YJ, Park S, Michelow IC. Co-seasonality and co-detection of respiratory
viruses and bacteraemia in children: a retrospective analysis. Clin Microbiol
Infect 2020;26(12):1690, e5-.e8.

21. Probst V, Spieker AJ, Stopczynski T, et al. Clinical Presentation and Severity of Adenovirus Detection Alone vs Adenovirus Co-detection With Other Respiratory Viruses in US Children With Acute Respiratory Illness from 2016 to 2018. J Pediatric Infect Dis Soc 2022;11(10):430–9.

22. Yanis A, Haddadin Z, Rahman H, et al. The Clinical Characteristics, Severity, and Seasonality of RSV Subtypes Among Hospitalized Children in Jordan. Pediatr Infect Dis J 2021;40(9):808–13.

23. Henrickson KJ, Hall CB. Diagnostic assays for respiratory syncytial virus disease. Pediatr Infect Dis J 2007;26(11 Suppl):S36–40.

24. Miernyk K, Bulkow L, DeByle C, et al. Performance of a rapid antigen test (Binax NOW® RSV) for diagnosis of respiratory syncytial virus compared with real-time polymerase chain reaction in a pediatric population. J Clin Virol 2011;50(3):240–3.

25. Dawood FS, Jara J, Estripeaut D, et al. What Is the Added Benefit of Oropharyngeal Swabs Compared to Nasal Swabs Alone for Respiratory Virus Detection in Hospitalized Children Aged <10 Years? J Infect Dis 2015;212(10):1600–3.

26. Firan M, Bawdon R, Radu C, et al. The MHC class I-related receptor, FcRn, plays an essential role in the maternofetal transfer of gamma-globulin in humans. Int Immunol 2001;13(8):993–1002.

27. Wilcox CR, Holder B, Jones CE. Factors Affecting the FcRn-Mediated Transplacental Transfer of Antibodies and Implications for Vaccination in Pregnancy. Front Immunol 2017;8:1294.

28. Chu HY, Tielsch J, Katz J, et al. Transplacental transfer of maternal respiratory syncytial virus (RSV) antibody and protection against RSV disease in infants in rural Nepal. J Clin Virol 2017;95:90–5.

29. JU Nyiro, Sande CJ, Mutunga M, et al. Absence of Association between Cord Specific Antibody Levels and Severe Respiratory Syncytial Virus (RSV) Disease in Early Infants: A Case Control Study from Coastal Kenya. PLoS One 2016;11(11):e0166706.

30. Capella C, Chaiwatpongsakorn S, Gorrell E, et al. Antibodies, and Disease Severity in Infants and Young Children With Acute Respiratory Syncytial Virus Infection. J Infect Dis 2017;216(11):1398–406.

31. Glezen WP, Paredes A, Allison JE, et al. Risk of respiratory syncytial virus infection for infants from low-income families in relationship to age, sex, ethnic group, and maternal antibody level. J Pediatr 1981;98(5):708–15.

32. Stensballe LG, Ravn H, Kristensen K, et al. Respiratory syncytial virus neutralizing antibodies in cord blood, respiratory syncytial virus hospitalization, and recurrent wheeze. J Allergy Clin Immunol 2009;123(2):398–403.

33. Updated guidance for palivizumab prophylaxis among infants and young children at increased risk of hospitalization for respiratory syncytial virus infection. Pediatrics 2014;134(2):e620–38.

34. Groothuis JR, Simoes EA, Levin MJ, et al. Prophylactic administration of respiratory syncytial virus immune globulin to high-risk infants and young children. The Respiratory Syncytial Virus Immune Globulin Study Group. N Engl J Med 1993;329(21):1524–30.

35. Finberg RW, Wang JP, Kurt-Jones EA. Toll like receptors and viruses. Rev Med Virol 2007;17(1):35–43.

36. Russell CD, Unger SA, Walton M, et al. The Human Immune Response to Respiratory Syncytial Virus Infection. Clin Microbiol Rev 2017;30(2):481–502.

37. Lotz MT, Peebles RS Jr. Mechanisms of respiratory syncytial virus modulation of airway immune responses. Curr Allergy Asthma Rep 2012;12(5):380–7.

38. Collins PL, Melero JA. Progress in understanding and controlling respiratory syncytial virus: still crazy after all these years. Virus Res 2011;162(1–2):80–99.
39. Falsey AR, Singh HK, Walsh EE. Serum antibody decay in adults following natural respiratory syncytial virus infection. J Med Virol 2006;78(11):1493–7.
40. Hall CB, Walsh EE, Long CE, et al. Immunity to and frequency of reinfection with respiratory syncytial virus. J Infect Dis 1991;163(4):693–8.
41. Walsh EE, Falsey AR. Humoral and mucosal immunity in protection from natural respiratory syncytial virus infection in adults. J Infect Dis 2004;190(2):373–8.
42. Bagga B, Cohelsky JE, Vaishnaw A, et al. Effect of Preexisting Serum and Mucosal Antibody on Experimental Respiratory Syncytial Virus (RSV) Challenge and Infection of Adults. J Infect Dis 2015;212(11):1719–25.
43. Habibi MS, Jozwik A, Makris S, et al. Impaired Antibody-mediated Protection and Defective IgA B-Cell Memory in Experimental Infection of Adults with Respiratory Syncytial Virus. Am J Respir Crit Care Med 2015;191(9):1040–9.
44. Welliver RC, Wong DT, Sun M, et al. The development of respiratory syncytial virus-specific IgE and the release of histamine in nasopharyngeal secretions after infection. N Engl J Med 1981;305(15):841–6.
45. Hall CB, Powell KR, MacDonald NE, et al. Respiratory syncytial viral infection in children with compromised immune function. N Engl J Med 1986;315(2):77–81.
46. Kim YJ, Boeckh M, Englund JA. Community respiratory virus infections in immunocompromised patients: hematopoietic stem cell and solid organ transplant recipients, and individuals with human immunodeficiency virus infection. Semin Respir Crit Care Med 2007;28(2):222–42.
47. Chi B, Dickensheets HL, Spann KM, et al. Alpha and lambda interferon together mediate suppression of CD4 T cells induced by respiratory syncytial virus. J Virol 2006;80(10):5032–40.
48. Graham BS, Rutigliano JA, Johnson TR. Respiratory syncytial virus immunobiology and pathogenesis. Virology 2002;297(1):1–7.
49. Kristjansson S, Bjarnarson SP, Wennergren G, et al. Respiratory syncytial virus and other respiratory viruses during the first 3 months of life promote a local TH2-like response. J Allergy Clin Immunol 2005;116(4):805–11.
50. Geevarghese B, Weinberg A. Cell-mediated immune responses to respiratory syncytial virus infection: magnitude, kinetics, and correlates with morbidity and age. Hum Vaccin Immunother 2014;10(4):1047–56.
51. Bloom-Feshbach K, Alonso WJ, Charu V, et al. Latitudinal variations in seasonal activity of influenza and respiratory syncytial virus (RSV): a global comparative review. PLoS One 2013;8(2):e54445.
52. Sloan C, Heaton M, Kang S, et al. The impact of temperature and relative humidity on spatiotemporal patterns of infant bronchiolitis epidemics in the contiguous United States. Health Place 2017;45:46–54.
53. Obando-Pacheco P, Justicia-Grande AJ, Rivero-Calle I, et al. Respiratory Syncytial Virus Seasonality: A Global Overview. J Infect Dis 2018;217(9):1356–64.
54. Stensballe LG, Devasundaram JK, Simoes EA. Respiratory syncytial virus epidemics: the ups and downs of a seasonal virus. Pediatr Infect Dis J 2003; 22(2 Suppl):S21–32.
55. Di Mattia G, Nenna R, Mancino E, et al. During the COVID-19 pandemic where has respiratory syncytial virus gone? Pediatr Pulmonol 2021;56(10):3106–9.
56. Liu L, Oza S, Hogan D, et al. Global, regional, and national causes of under-5 mortality in 2000-15: an updated systematic analysis with implications for the Sustainable Development Goals. Lancet 2016;388(10063):3027–35.

57. Li Y, Wang X, Blau DM, et al. Global, regional, and national disease burden estimates of acute lower respiratory infections due to respiratory syncytial virus in children younger than 5 years in 2019: a systematic analysis. Lancet 2022; 399(10340):2047–64.

58. Esposito S, Abu Raya B, Baraldi E, et al. RSV Prevention in All Infants: Which Is the Most Preferable Strategy? Front Immunol 2022;13:880368.

59. Mazur NI, Higgins D, Nunes MC, et al. The respiratory syncytial virus vaccine landscape: lessons from the graveyard and promising candidates. Lancet Infect Dis 2018;18(10):e295–311.

60. Shi T, Vennard S, Jasiewicz F, et al. Disease Burden Estimates of Respiratory Syncytial Virus related Acute Respiratory Infections in Adults With Comorbidity: A Systematic Review and Meta-Analysis. J Infect Dis 2022;226(Suppl 1): S17–21.

61. Savic M, Penders Y, Shi T, et al. Respiratory syncytial virus disease burden in adults aged 60 years and older in high-income countries: A systematic literature review and meta-analysis. Influenza Other Respir Viruses 2023;17(1):e13031.

62. Glezen WP, Taber LH, Frank AL, et al. Risk of primary infection and reinfection with respiratory syncytial virus. Am J Dis Child 1986;140(6):543–6.

63. McLaurin KK, Farr AM, Wade SW, et al. Respiratory syncytial virus hospitalization outcomes and costs of full-term and preterm infants. J Perinatol 2016; 36(11):990–6.

64. Martinello RA, Chen MD, Weibel C, et al. Correlation between respiratory syncytial virus genotype and severity of illness. J Infect Dis 2002;186(6):839–42.

65. Garg I, Shekhar R, Sheikh AB, et al. Impact of COVID-19 on the Changing Patterns of Respiratory Syncytial Virus Infections. Infect Dis Rep 2022;14(4): 558–68.

66. Centers for Disease Control and Prevention. RSV National Trends: cdc.gov. 2023 [updated January 18, 2023. Available at: https://www.cdc.gov/surveillance/nrevss/rsv/natl-trend.html.

67. Smith DK, Seales S, Budzik C. Respiratory Syncytial Virus Bronchiolitis in Children. Am Fam Physician 2017;95(2):94–9.

68. Heikkinen T, Thint M, Chonmaitree T. Prevalence of various respiratory viruses in the middle ear during acute otitis media. N Engl J Med 1999;340(4):260–4.

69. Fauroux B, Simões EAF, Checchia PA, et al. The Burden and Long-term Respiratory Morbidity Associated with Respiratory Syncytial Virus Infection in Early Childhood. Infect Dis Ther 2017;6(2):173–97.

70. Zomer-Kooijker K, van der Ent CK, Ermers MJ, et al. Increased risk of wheeze and decreased lung function after respiratory syncytial virus infection. PLoS One 2014;9(1):e87162.

71. Chu HY, Katz J, Tielsch J, et al. Clinical Presentation and Birth Outcomes Associated with Respiratory Syncytial Virus Infection in Pregnancy. PLoS One 2016; 11(3):e0152015.

72. Wheeler SM, Dotters-Katz S, Heine RP, et al. Maternal Effects of Respiratory Syncytial Virus Infection during Pregnancy. Emerg Infect Dis 2015;21(11): 1951–5.

73. Hause AM, Avadhanula V, Maccato ML, et al. Clinical characteristics and outcomes of respiratory syncytial virus infection in pregnant women. Vaccine 2019;37(26):3464–71.

74. Falsey AR, Hennessey PA, Formica MA, et al. Respiratory syncytial virus infection in elderly and high-risk adults. N Engl J Med 2005;352(17):1749–59.

75. Delahoy MJ, Whitaker M, O'Halloran A, et al. Characteristics and Maternal and Birth Outcomes of Hospitalized Pregnant Women with Laboratory-Confirmed COVID-19 - COVID-NET, 13 States, March 1-August 22, 2020. MMWR Morb Mortal Wkly Rep 2020;69(38):1347–54.
76. Håberg SE, Trogstad L, Gunnes N, et al. Risk of fetal death after pandemic influenza virus infection or vaccination. N Engl J Med 2013;368(4):333–40.
77. Thompson WW, Shay DK, Weintraub E, et al. Mortality associated with influenza and respiratory syncytial virus in the United States. JAMA 2003;289(2):179–86.
78. Branche AR, Falsey AR. Respiratory syncytial virus infection in older adults: an under-recognized problem. Drugs Aging 2015;32(4):261–9.
79. Falsey AR, Walsh EE, Looney RJ, et al. Comparison of respiratory syncytial virus humoral immunity and response to infection in young and elderly adults. J Med Virol 1999;59(2):221–6.
80. Renaud C, Campbell AP. Changing epidemiology of respiratory viral infections in hematopoietic cell transplant recipients and solid organ transplant recipients. Curr Opin Infect Dis 2011;24(4):333–43.
81. Zamora MR, Budev M, Rolfe M, et al. RNA interference therapy in lung transplant patients infected with respiratory syncytial virus. Am J Respir Crit Care Med 2011;183(4):531–8.
82. American Academy of Pediatrics Committee on Infectious Diseases. Use of ribavirin in the treatment of respiratory syncytial virus infection. Pediatrics 1993;92(3):501–4.
83. Everard ML, Swarbrick A, Rigby AS, et al. The effect of ribavirin to treat previously healthy infants admitted with acute bronchiolitis on acute and chronic respiratory morbidity. Respir Med 2001;95(4):275–80.
84. Domachowske JB, Anderson EJ, Goldstein M. The Future of Respiratory Syncytial Virus Disease Prevention and Treatment. Infect Dis Ther 2021;10(Suppl 1): 47–60.
85. Chemaly RF, Aitken SL, Wolfe CR, et al. Aerosolized ribavirin: the most expensive drug for pneumonia. Transpl Infect Dis 2016;18(4):634–6.
86. Sinclair SM, Jones JK, Miller RK, et al. Final results from the ribavirin pregnancy registry, 2004-2020. Birth Defects Res 2022;114(20):1376–91.
87. Rodriguez-Fernandez R, Mejias A, Ramilo O. Monoclonal Antibodies for Prevention of Respiratory Syncytial Virus Infection. Pediatr Infect Dis J 2021;40(5s): S35–9.
88. Ralston SL, Lieberthal AS, Meissner HC, et al. Clinical Practice Guideline: The Diagnosis, Management, and Prevention of Bronchiolitis. Pediatrics 2014; 134(5):e1474–502.
89. Palivizumab. a humanized respiratory syncytial virus monoclonal antibody, reduces hospitalization from respiratory syncytial virus infection in high-risk infants. The IMpact-RSV Study Group. Pediatrics 1998;102(3 Pt 1):531–7.
90. Nirsevimab AstraZeneca. US regulatory submission accepted for the prevention of RSV lower respiratory tract disease in infants and children up to age 24 months 2023 [updated 5 January 2023. Available at: https://www.astrazeneca.com/media-centre/press-releases/2023/nirsevimab-us-regulatory-submission-accepted-for-the-prevention-of-rsv-lower-respiratory-tract-disease-in-infants-and-children.html.
91. Hammitt LL, Dagan R, Yuan Y, et al. Nirsevimab for Prevention of RSV in Healthy Late-Preterm and Term Infants. N Engl J Med 2022;386(9):837–46.
92. PATH. RSV Vaccine and mAb Snapshot: path.org; 2023 [updated 3 January 2023. Available at: https://media.path.org/documents/RSV-Snapshot_03J

AN2023_HighResolution.pdfl=1*9bwa7b*_gcl_aw*R0NMLjE2NzU1NTkxODY
uQ2owS0NRaUF0NjZlQmhDbkFSSXNBS2YzWk5FNnQxNm81LW1sR2tLY1-
d6U05QQ0Z0a2o3a3EtU014VHZXUzMtTWMtMW8yNzhrQjBFFWXkyZ2FBcH-
pYRUFMd193Y0l.*_ga*NDE1NTM2MzcuMTY3NDMyNTQ0OA..*_ga_YBSE7Z
KDQM*MTY3NTYyNDg0NS45LjEuMTY3NTYyNTA2OC4wLjAuMA.

93. Kachikis A, Eckert LO, Englund J. Who's the Target: Mother or Baby? Viral Immunol 2018;31(2):184–94.

94. Munoz FM. Respiratory syncytial virus in infants: is maternal vaccination a realistic strategy? Curr Opin Infect Dis 2015;28(3):221–4.

95. Skoff TH, Deng L, Bozio CH, et al. US Infant Pertussis Incidence Trends Before and After Implementation of the Maternal Tetanus, Diphtheria, and Pertussis Vaccine. JAMA Pediatr 2023. https://doi.org/10.1001/jamapediatrics.2022.5689.

96. Madhi SA, Polack FP, Piedra PA, et al. Respiratory Syncytial Virus Vaccination during Pregnancy and Effects in Infants. N Engl J Med 2020;383(5):426–39.

97. Larkin H. Investigational RSV Vaccine Given During Pregnancy Protects Newborns. JAMA 2022;328(22):2201.

98. Mireku A. Race to the finish: pharma edges closer to approval with RSV vaccines: Pharmaceutical Technology. 2023 [updated 1 February 2023. Available at: https://www.pharmaceutical-technology.com/features/race-to-the-finish-pharma-edges-closer-to-approval-with-rsv-vaccines/.

99. Karron RA, Buchholz UJ, Collins PL. Live-attenuated respiratory syncytial virus vaccines. Curr Top Microbiol Immunol 2013;372:259–84.

100. Karron RA, Luongo C, Thumar B, et al. A gene deletion that up-regulates viral gene expression yields an attenuated RSV vaccine with improved antibody responses in children. Sci Transl Med 2015;7(312):312ra175.

Moving?

Make sure your subscription moves with you!

To notify us of your new address, find your **Clinics Account Number** (located on your mailing label above your name), and contact customer service at:

Email: journalscustomerservice-usa@elsevier.com

800-654-2452 (subscribers in the U.S. & Canada)
314-447-8871 (subscribers outside of the U.S. & Canada)

Fax number: 314-447-8029

Elsevier Health Sciences Division
Subscription Customer Service
3251 Riverport Lane
Maryland Heights, MO 63043

*To ensure uninterrupted delivery of your subscription, please notify us at least 4 weeks in advance of move.